CARDIOLOGY RESEARCH AND CLINICAL DEVELOPMENTS

CORONARY COMPUTED TOMOGRAPHY ANGIOGRAPHY IN CORONARY ARTERY DISEASE

A SYSTEMATIC REVIEW OF IMAGE QUALITY, DIAGNOSTIC ACCURACY AND RADIATION DOSE

CARDIOLOGY RESEARCH AND CLINICAL DEVELOPMENTS

Additional books in this series can be found on Nova's website under the Series tab.

Additional E-books in this series can be found on Nova's website under the E-book tab.

MEDICAL PROCEDURES, TESTING AND TECHNOLOGY

Additional books in this series can be found on Nova's website under the Series tab.

Additional E-books in this series can be found on Nova's website under the E-book tab.

CARDIOLOGY RESEARCH AND CLINICAL DEVELOPMENTS

CORONARY COMPUTED TOMOGRAPHY ANGIOGRAPHY IN CORONARY ARTERY DISEASE

A SYSTEMATIC REVIEW OF IMAGE QUALITY, DIAGNOSTIC ACCURACY AND RADIATION DOSE

ZHONGHUA SUN

NOVA BIOMEDICAL

New York

For permission to use material from this book please contact us:
Telephone 631-231-7269; Fax 631-231-8175
Web Site: http://www.novapublishers.com

Library of Congress Cataloging-in-Publication Data

Library of Congress Control Number: 2012954499
ISBN: 978-1-62417-604-3

Published by Nova Science Publishers, Inc. † New York

Contents

Preface

Coronary artery disease is the leading cause of death in the developed countries and it is becoming increasingly common in the developing world. Conventional invasive coronary angiography currently remains the gold standard for the evaluation of patients with known or suspected coronary artery disease. Limitations of the modality include its invasiveness, expense, and time consumption, with small but substantial procedure-related complications. This indicates the necessity and importance of identifying a reliable non-invasive imaging modality for detection and diagnosis of coronary artery disease.

Computed tomography (CT) has become a widely used non-invasive imaging modality for the diagnosis of cardiovascular disease since the advent of spiral CT in early 1990s. However, diagnostic applications of CT in cardiac imaging with single-slice CT scanners were limited due to restrictions in spatial and temporal resolution. The introduction of multislice CT scanners in 1998 represented another significant advancement in CT technology, and for the first time CT angiography with ECG-gating is able to acquire cardiac images at considerably faster volume coverage with improved spatial and temporal resolution. Since then, multislice CT angiography in cardiac imaging (which is nowadays called coronary CT angiography) has become increasingly used for the diagnosis of coronary artery disease. With the wide availability of dual-source CT and the recent introduction of 320-slice CT the diagnostic accuracy of coronary CT angiography has been significantly enhanced, thus, the spectrum of coronary CT angiography in cardiac imaging will be expanded in the near future.

Over the last decade studies on coronary CT angiography have been increasingly published in the literature with a focus on the diagnostic performance of coronary CT angiography in the diagnosis of coronary artery disease. This is mainly due to the high spatial and temporal resolution which is available with the latest multislice CT scanners. However, it is important for researchers and clinicians to be aware of the variable results reported in these studies with regard to the diagnostic value and study limitations due to heterogeneity of study design and patient selection. Judicious use of coronary CT angiography in routine clinical practice is an evidence-based practice, which can be addressed by a systematic review of the literature. This book fulfills this goal.

This book is intended to fill the gap by providing a systematic review and meta-analysis of the diagnostic value, image quality and radiation dose of coronary CT angiography. It serves as a comprehensive piece of literature that encompasses all aspects from the technical principles of coronary CT angiography image acquisition to clinical diagnostic value and potential pitfalls of cardiac CT imaging. The primary motion to write this book is to provide an overview of the current status of coronary CT angiography in coronary artery disease with a focus on the diagnostic value, image quality and radiation dose, as well as the current research directions of this fast evolving technique. Effects of various scanning parameters on radiation dose and image quality are also addressed in detail.

The book consists of 13 chapters covering various topics related to the coronary CT angiography with inclusion of comprehensive recently published literature. Chapter 1 is an introduction of the coronary artery disease with a focus on the increased application of coronary CT angiography in clinical diagnosis. Chapter 2 describes the imaging principles of cardiac imaging and technical developments of coronary CT angiography including a variety of reconstructed visualizations. Chapter 3 discusses the radiation dose measurements in cardiac CT and strategies for dose reduction. Commonly used or recommended approaches for coronary CT angiography dose reduction are discussed in detail. Chapters 4, 5, 6 and 10 focus entirely on the systematic review and meta-analysis of diagnostic value of coronary CT angiography performed with 64-slice CT, dual-source CT, 320-slice CT, and coronary CT angiography with use of prospective ECG-triggering, respectively. Chapter 7 presents a systematic review of the research directions in coronary CT angiography based on analysis of the articles published in five top radiology journals over the last 6 years. Chapter 8 compares retrospectively ECG-gated with prospectively ECG-triggered coronary CT angiography in terms of diagnostic value and radiation dose, while chapter 9 elucidates the effectiveness of prospectively ECG-triggered coronary CT angiography in terms of diagnostic accuracy when compared to invasive coronary angiography. Chapter 11 discusses how coronary CT angiography can be used wisely by clinicians and when it should be requested and how its benefits can be maximized from a clinical perspective. Chapter 12 describes the current status of coronary CT angiography and challenges with regard to the utilization of this fast growing technique. Finally, chapter 13 is a brief summary and conclusion of coronary CT angiography.

This book is intended primarily for radiologists, cardiologists and medical imaging technologists who are actively involved in performing coronary CT angiography examinations. However, other physicians, residents, postgraduate students and other healthcare professions who are dealing with cardiac imaging could also benefit from it. This book can also be used as guidance for radiology residents or postgraduate students to conduct systematic review or meta-analysis as part of the research training program or research degree. I hope this book will improve understanding of the diagnostic performance of coronary CT angiography and it will contribute considerably to the judicious use of coronary CT angiography in the diagnosis of coronary artery disease.

Zhonghua Sun, MB, PhD

Chapter 1

Introduction

Coronary artery disease (CAD) is one of the leading causes of morbidity and mortality in most developed countries and its prevalence is increasing in developing countries. Conventional invasive coronary angiography still remains the gold standard in the diagnosis of patients with known or suspected CAD [1]. However, this conventional modality suffers from some limitations including its invasiness, expense, time consumption, with a small but substantial complication rate (stroke, coronary artery dissection, cardiac arrhythmias, hemorrhage at the arteriotomy site, and pseudoaneurysm formation) [2]. The overall complication rate associated with invasive coronary angiography is reported to be about 1.8% [3]. The mortality rate from the procedure is 0.1%, but may be up to 0.55% in patients with co-morbid medical conditions [4]. Furthermore, invasive coronary angiography usually requires a short hospital stay and causes discomfort for the patients. It is reported that only one-third of all invasive coronary angiography examinations in the United States are performed in conjunction with an interventional procedure, while the rest are performed only for diagnostic purposes, which is only for verification of the presence and degree of CAD [5]. Therefore, a non-invasive technique for imaging of the coronary artery disease is highly desirable.

Cardiac imaging has always been technically challenging due to the heart's continuous movement. Traditionally, noninvasive cardiac imaging was dominated by electron-beam computed tomography (EBCT) [6, 7]. Morphological assessment of cardiac strucures became possible with EBCT due to its high temporal resolution (50-100 ms) and use of prospective eletrocardiographic (ECG) triggering. EBCT with prospective ECG triggering was mainly applied in the detection and evaluation of calcification in the coronary arteries (coronary calcium scoring), which is considered a risk indicator of the degree and severity of CAD, thus, is commonly used for risk stratification in asymptomatic patients [8, 9]. Higher coronary artery calcium scores were associated with increased plaque burden and increased cardiovascular risk [9, 10]. EBCT had limited value in the detection of coronary stenosis due to its inferior spatial resolution (1.5 mm to 3.0 mm in longitudinal direction), thus, it was not promoted as a means to identify the presence of coronary stenoses. Imaging of the heart has moved into the diagnostic era with the introduction of multislice CT (MSCT) angiography and development of electrocardiography-synchronized scanning and reconstruction techniques [11-13], leading to the widely application of coronary CT angiography examinations across the world.

Coronary CT angiography has been well established as a valuable diagnostic modality in the detection of coronary artery disease for more than a decade. The rapid technology evolution from early generation of 4-slice CT to the latest dual-source CT and 320-slice scanners has yielded dramatic improvements in spatial and temporal resolution [14]. Improvement of image quality has been reported in the visualization of all coronary artery branches with high sensitivity and specificity achieved [15-17]. As a result, there is a growing interest in using cardiac CT for evaluation of the heart for many conditions. Coronary CT angiography is not only applied to detect and quantify the coronary artery calcifications, but also is used to image the coronary vasculature, diagnose the degree of coronary stenosis and assess the myocardium [14]. Coronary CT angiography is a recently recommended term used to describe the specific application of MSCT imaging in the diagnosis of CAD. The potential to visualize coronary remodeling and plaques non-invasively enables this technique to be used as a key imaging modality towards CAD [18, 19].

There have been many studies reported on the use of coronary CT angiography in the diagnosis of coronary artery stenosis as a potential alternative to invasive coronary angiography. A huge amount of literature has been published on this technique, with increasing evidence claiming that coronary CT angiography serves as a reliable less-invasive modality in selected patients. The purpose of this book is to examine the currently available literature on coronary CT angiography and to use this for evaluation of the technical and diagnostic performance of coronary CT angiography.

The following chapters in this book will provide an overview of the diagnostic value of coronary CT angiography in CAD, with a focus on the diagnostic performance of 64- and more slice CT angiography, based on a systematic review and meta-analysis of the evidences that are available in the literature. A recently developed protocol, prospective ECG-triggering will be discussed in detail with regard to the diagnostic performance and radiation dose, and research directions and challenges of coronary CT angiography will be highlighted as well.

References

[1] Becker CR. Assessment of coronary arteries with CT. *Radiol Clin North Am* 2002;40:773–782.

[2] Heffernan EJ, Dodd JD, Malone DE. Cardiac multidetector CT: technical and diagnostic evaluation with evidence-based practice techniques. *Radiology* 2008; 248: 336-377.

[3] Hoffmann MH, Shi H, Schmitz BL, et al. Noninvasive coronary angiography with multislice computed tomography. *JAMA* 2005;293: 2471–2478.

[4] Johnson LW, Lozner EC, Johnson S, et al. Coronary arteriography 1984–1987: a report of the Registry of the Society for Cardiac Angiography and Interventions. I. Results and complications. *Cathet Cardiovasc Diagn* 1989; 17:5–10.

[5] American Heart Association, American Stroke Association. 2002 *Heart and stroke statistical update*. Dallas, TX: The American Heart Association, 2002.

[6] Rumberger JA, Sheedy PF 2nd, Breen JF, Fitzpatrick LA, Schwartz RS. Electron beam computed tomography and coronary artery disease: scanning for coronary artery calcification. *Mayo Clin Proc* 1996;71:369-77.
[7] Keelan PC, Bielak LF, Ashai K, et al. Long-term prognostic value of coronary calcification detected by electron beam computed tomography in patients undergoing coronary angiography. *Circulation* 2001 Jul;104(4):412-7.
[8] Arad Y, Goodman KJ, Roth M, Newstein D, Guerci D. Coronary calcification, coronary disease risk factors, C-reactive protein, and atherosclerotic cardiovascular disease events: the St. Francis Heart Study. *J Am Coll Cardiol* 2005; 46: 158-165.
[9] Hecht HS, Budoff MJ, Berman DS, Ehrlich J, Rumberger JA. Coronary artery calcium scanning: clinical paradigms for cardiac riskk assessment and treatment. *Am Heart J* 2006; 151: 1139-1146.
[10] Haberl R, Becker A, Leber A, et al. Correlation of coronary calcification and angiographically documented sgtenoses in patients with suspected coronary artery disease: results of 1,764 patients. *J Am Coll Cardiol* 2001; 37: 451-457.
[11] McCollough CH, Zink FE. Performance evaluation of a multi-slice CT system. *Med Phys* 1999; 26: 2223-2230.
[12] Hu H, He HD, Foley WD, et al. Four multidetector-row helical CT: image quality and volume coverage speed. *Radiology* 2000; 215: 55-62.
[13] Nieman K, Oudkerk M, Rensing BJ, et al. Coronary angiography with multi-slice computed tomography. *Lancet* 2001; 357: 599-603.
[14] Sun Z, Choo GH, Ng KH. Coronary CT angiography: current status and continuing challenges. *Br J Radiol* 2012; 85: 495-510.
[15] Pugliese F, Mollet NR, Runza G, et al. Diagnostic accuracy of non-invasive 64-slice CT coronary angiography in patients with stable angina pectoris. *Eur Radiol* 2006;16:575–82.
[16] Ong TK, Chin SP, Liew CK, et al. Accuracy of 64-row multidetector computed tomography in detecting coronary artery disease in 134 symptomatic patients: influence of calcification. *Am Heart J* 2006;151:1323. e 1-6.
[17] Raff GL, Gallagher MJ, O'Neill WW, Goldstein JA. Diagnostic accuracy of non-invasive coronary angiography using 64-slice spiral computed tomography. *J Am Coll Cardiol* 2005;46:552–557.
[18] Kunimasa T, Sato Y, Sugi K, Mori M. Evaluation by multislice computed tomography of atherosclerotic coronary artery plaques in non-culprit, remote coronary arteries of patients with acute coronary syndrome. *Circ J* 2005; 69: 1346-1351.
[19] Achenbach S, Ropers D, Hoffmann U, et al. Assessment of coronary remodeling in stenotic and nonstenotic coronary atherosclerotic lesions by multidetector spiral computed tomography. *J Am Coll Cardiol* 2004; 43: 842-847.

Chapter 2

Coronary CT Angiography: Imaging Principles and Technical Developments

Abstract

Multislice CT has undergone rapid technical developments over the last decade, and the most important application of multislice CT imaging is coronary CT angiography with its widespread application in cardiac imaging. Imaging of coronary arteries is technically challenging because of its small vessel diameters, tortuous path around the myocardium and continuous motion of the heart during cardiac scans.

Thus, high spatial and temporal resolution of coronary CT angiography is essential to ensure acquisition of motion-free cardiac images. In addition, specific scanning protocols are developed for coronary CT angiography to minimize the artefacts resulting from cardiac motion. This chapter focuses on the technical details of coronary CT angiography, and presents information about the technical developments of multislice CT scanners from early generation of 4-slice to the recent models of 320-slice CT.

Keywords: Coronary artery, coronary CT angiography, electrocardiographic gating, multislice CT, reconstruction

2.1. Coronary Artery Tree-Anatomical Details

Normal coronary artery diameter has been established with invasive coronary angiography. The average size varies with gender (approximately 3 mm in females and 4 mm in males) [1]. The four main coronary arteries evaluated at cardiac CT are right coronary artery (RCA), left main stem, left anterior descending (LAD) and left circumflex (LCx). The coronary arteries are evaluated according to the American Heart Association (AHA) classification system, which divides the coronary arteries into 15-segment [2]. Figure 2.1 shows the 15 coronary segments arising from these four main coronary arteries.

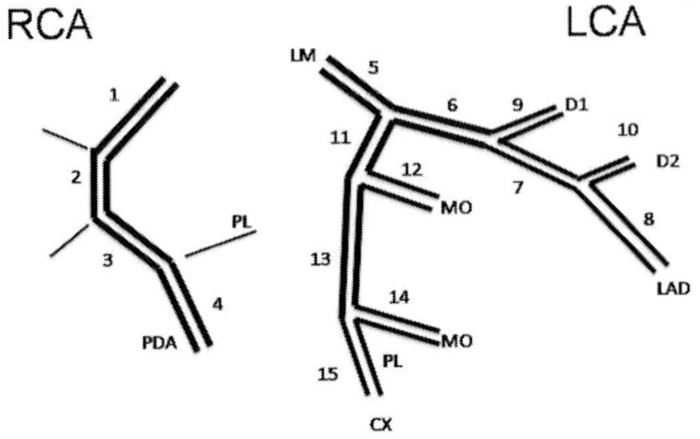

Figure 2.1. Classification of coronary segments is performed by dividing the coronary tree into 15 segments (modified from the American Heart Association [2]). Segments 1-4 correspond to right coronary artery (RCA); segment 5, to the left main stem; segments 6-10 to the left coronary artery (LCA); segments 11-15 to the left circumflex (LCX). MO-marginal branch, D1-first diagonal branch, D2-second diagonal branch, PL-posterolateral branch, PDA-posterior descending artery.

2.1.1. Left Coronary Artery

The left coronary artery (LCA) normally arises from the left aortic sinus and passes to the left between pulmonary trunk and left atrium to reach the coronary groove. It courses for a variable distance before giving rise to the LAD and the LCx from the short branch of LCA, the left main stem (Figure 2.2).

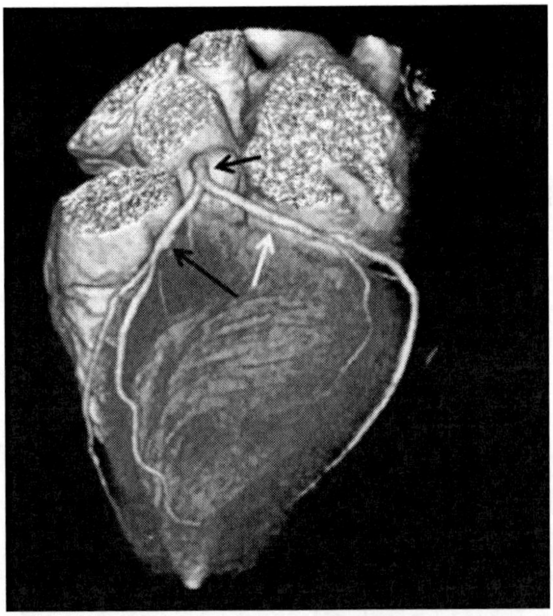

Figure 2.2. Volume rendering image shows the LCA (short black arrow) arising from the aorta and bifurcating into the proximal LAD (long black arrow) and the proximal LCx artery (white arrow).

The LAD artery courses anterolaterally in the epicardial fat of the anterior interventricular groove and provides blood supply to the majority of the left ventricle (Figure 2.3). The major branches are the diagonal and septal perforating arteries [3, 4]. The LCx artery is another major branch of the LCA. It courses in the left atrioventricular groove, giving rise to obtuse marginal branches (Figure 2.4).

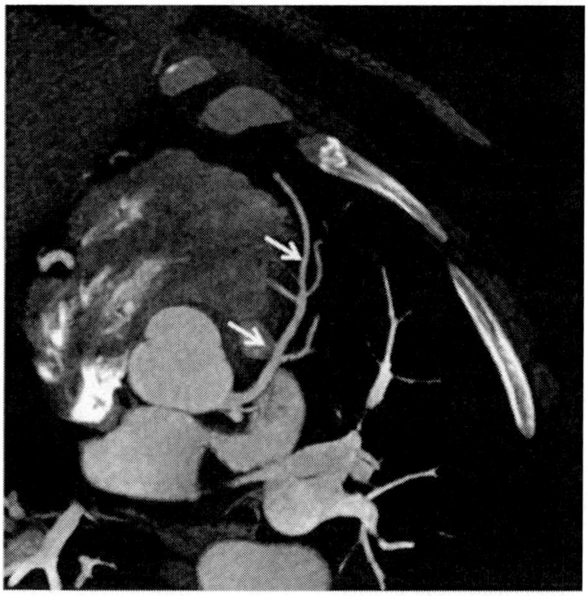

a

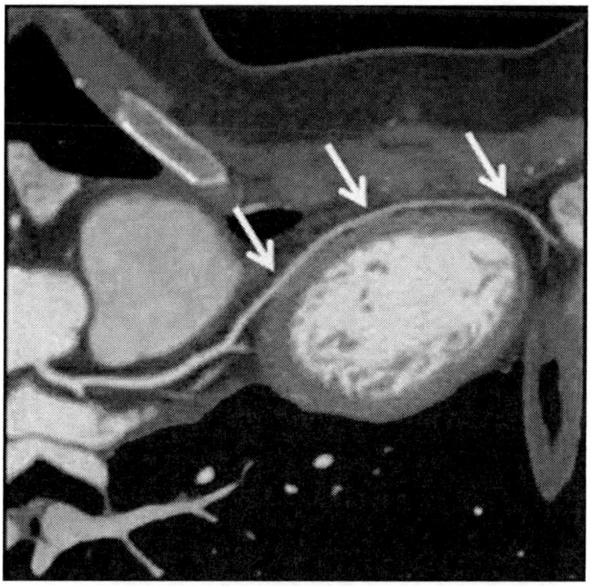

b

Figure 2.3. Oblique axial (A) and vertical long-axis (B) multiplanar reformation (MPR) images show the normal LAD artery (arrows) coursing in the epicardial fat of the interventricular groove toward the left ventricle apex.

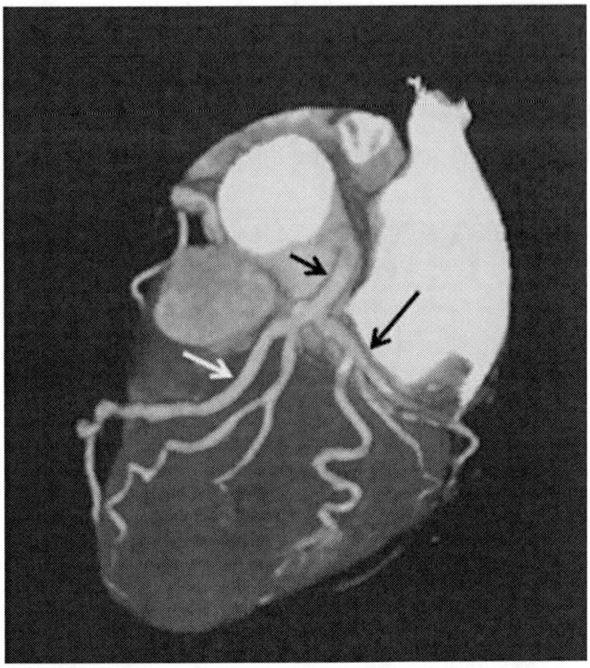

Figure 2.4. Volume rendering image shows the left main stem (show black arrow) divides into the LCx (long black arrow) and LAD (white arrow) arteries.

In approximately 15% of patients, a third branch, ramus intermedius (RI) branch, arises at the bifurcation of the LCA, leading to a trifurcation (Figure 2.5) [5]. The RI branch's course is similar to that of a diagonal branch of the LAD artery, which courses laterally toward the left ventricle free wall.

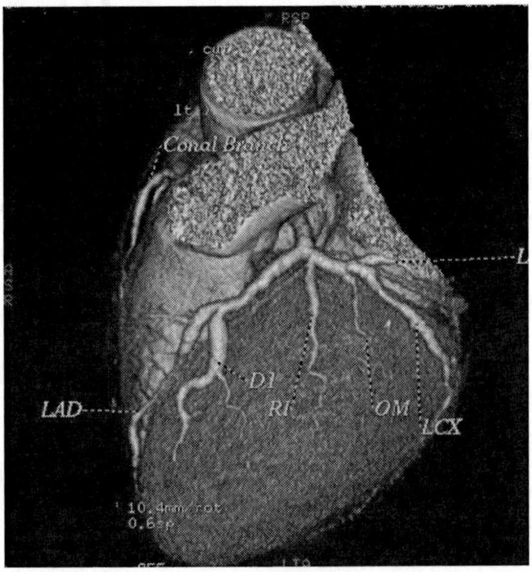

Figure 2.5. Volume rendering image shows the ramus intermedius (RI) branch arising between the LAD and LCx arteries, resulting in a trifurcation of the LCA. D1-first diagonal branch, OM-obtuse marginal branch.

2.1.2. Right Coronary Artery

The RCA normally arises from the right coronary sinus or the root of the aorta, and courses in the right atrioventricular groove toward the crux of the heart. In approximately 50-60% of patients, the first branch of the RCA is a conus artery (Figure 2.6). Multiple ventricular branches arise from the RCA, with the largest being the acute marginal branch [4].

The coronary artery that gives rise to the posterior descending artery (PDA) and posterolateral branch is referred to as the "dominance" artery. The RCA is dominant in about 70% of cases (Figure 2.7), while the LCA is dominant in approximately 10% of cases, and in the remaining cases, the RCA and LCA are codominant.

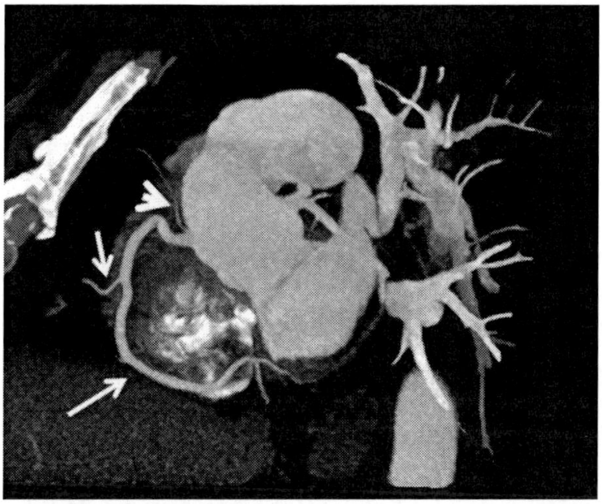

Figure 2.6. Coronal maximum-intensity projection (MIP) shows the conus artery (arrowhead) arising from the RCA (long white arrow). Short white arrow indicates the acute marginal branch.

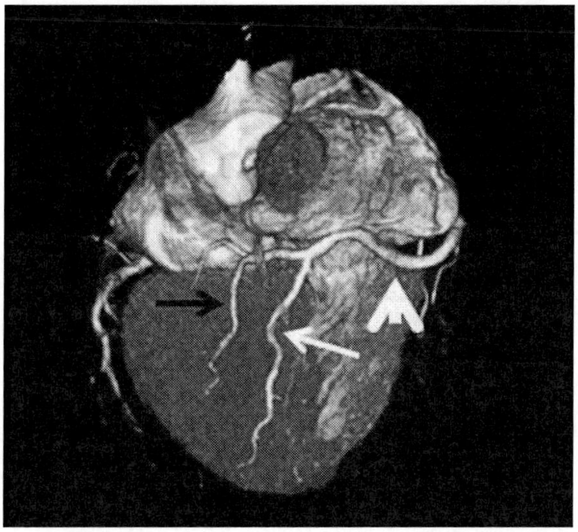

Figure 2.7. Volume rendering image shows the inferior surface of the heart. A right-dominant system is depicted, with the PDA (white arrow) arising from the RCA (arrowhead). A posterolateral branch (black arrow) is also noted.

2.2. Cardiac Imaging Principles

Imaging of a moving organ such as heart requires dedicated approaches that result in decreased motion artefacts by either scanning or reconstructing raw data at the point of least cardiac motion. In cardiac CT, there are two well-established modes for imaging the constantly moving heart and coronary arteries: prospective electrocardiography (ECG)-triggering and retrospective ECG-gating [5].

2.2.1. Spatial and Temporal Resolution

The demand from cardiac CT is that images must be acquired with high spatial resolution, high temporal resolution, and true volume datasets. Thus, the aim of cardiac CT is to develop advanced scanners which provide super-fast gantry rotation times, submillimetre slice thickness and datasets consisting of hundreds of thin slices with postprocessing allowing isotropic reconstruction in any plane.

Spatial resolution determines the ability of an imaging technique to visualize contours of small structures within the scanned volume. High spatial resolution is essential to enable visualization of small coronary arteries and plaques and delineation of complex cardiac anatomy with excellent diagnostic quality. Improvement of spatial resolution in cardiac CT is of particular importance for the evaluation of coronary artery calcium and diagnostic performance of coronary CT angiography. Many cardiac structures, especially the coronary arteries and the cardiac valves including the valve flaps, represent small and complex 3D structures that require very high and submillimeter isotropic spatial resolution with longitudinal resolution close or equal to in-plane resolution (0.4-0.6 mm) [6]. The lumen diameter of the main segments of the coronary artery tree ranges from 3-5 mm in the main segments to about 1 mm in the distal segments. Detection and quantification of coronary artery stenosis with the ability to distinguish a minimal 20% change in the diameter of the vessel lumen for the larger-caliber vessels represents a viable goal for cardiac CT imaging. To achieve this, CT scanners need to provide a spatial resolution in all three dimensions (isotropic voxel along x, y and x-axes) of at least 0.5 mm for visualization of the main coronary vessels and of smaller branches [6]. Thus, in-plane and through-plane resolution well below 1 mm are needed to accurately assess the main coronary segments, including lumen narrowing and plaques.

With early type of multislice CT scanners such as 4-slice CT, the image quality was suboptimal because of relatively limited spatial resolution (0.6 x 0.6 x 1.0 mm) as well as the long duration of the required breath-hold (as long as 40 s), thus, the unassessable segments could be as high as 30% in studies performed with 4-slice scanners [7]. With the introduction of 16-slice (0.5 x 0.5 x 0.6 mm) [8] and development of 64-slice CT, acquisition of isotropic volume data is made available, especially with 64-slice CT (0.5 x 0.5 x 0.5 mm), thus detection of main coronary artery and side branches is significantly improved when compared to earlier types of multislice CT scanners [7, 9]. Although spatial resolution of coronary CT angiography is improving, it is inherently inferior to that of invasive coronary angiography (0.1-0.2 mm).

Temporal resolution is the amount of time it takes to acquire the necessary scan data to reconstruct an image [10]. High temporal resolution is critical to minimize or eliminate motion artefacts associated with the beating heart to make it possible to image the entire heart volume in a single breath-hold. Improved temporal resolution in cardiac CT is achieved by fast data acquisition (fast rotation of the X-ray tube), but even more importantly by a dedicated reconstruction algorithm [11]. The temporal resolution of multislice CT scanners is essentially determined by the speed of gantry rotation. As it is possible to accurately reconstruct images using data acquired from a 180 degree rotation rather than the full 360 degree rotation, the temporal resolution is equal to half the gantry rotation speed (e.g. 250 ms for 500-ms rotation time, and 200 ms for 400-ms rotation time). In all modern multislice CT scanners, the half-scan reconstruction technique is the method of choice for image reconstruction in cardiac CT applications. In clinical applications, the heart should be sufficiently centered within the scan field of view in order to maintain a consistent and stable temporal resolution of about half the rotation time [6].

A temporal resolution of less than 250 ms is sufficient for motion-free imaging in the diastolic phase for heart rates less than 60 beats per minute (bpm), whereas a temporal resolution of 50 ms is needed in the systolic phase imaging. With increases in heart rates, higher temporal resolution is required [12]. A temporal resolution of less than 200 ms is required for heart rates less than 70 bpm, and approximately 150 ms for clinically usual heart rates up to 90 bpm [6]. It can be expected that a temporal resolution of about 100 ms is sufficient for imaging the heart during the diastolic or end-systolic phase also at higher heart rates [13]. The temporal resolution for 4-slice CT is 250 ms (gantry rotation is 500 ms), and this is further improved to 165 ms for 16- and 64-slice CT, and to 83 ms for dual-source CT [14, 15]. In comparison, invasive coronary angiography has an excellent temporal resolution, which is less than 20 ms. Studies using dual-source CT showed promising results with high diagnostic accuracy for detection of coronary artery disease, and most importantly the image quality is less dependent on heart rates [16-18].

Although temporal resolution with coronary CT angiography depends on several factors related to the inherent characteristics of the CT scanner (gantry rotation time, number of detector rows, etc), appropriate utilization of ECG-gating and the type of synchronization algorithm is of paramount importance and comprises an essential component of cardiac CT imaging. ECG-gating and synchronization allows data acquisition and image reconstruction at specific segments or points in the cardiac cycle, thus, optimizing image quality while determining the type of information available to clinical diagnosis. There are currently two methods of ECG-gating, namely, prospective ECG-triggering and retrospective ECG-gating.

2.2.2. Retrospective ECG-gating

A retrospective ECG-gating technique is used in the spiral mode. In the spiral mode, the CT data is acquired continuously while the table (and the patient) moves simultaneously at a constant speed (Figure 2.8). Retrospectively ECG-gated CT angiography of the heart requires a highly overlapping spiral scan with a spiral table speed adapted to the heart rate to ensure complete phase-consistent coverage of the heart with overlapping image sections. Using this technique, data is acquired throughout the entire cardiac cycle at a very low pitch (0.2-0.4) while simultaneously recording the patient's ECG signal. On the basis of patient's ECG, only a small part of the raw data is used for image reconstruction to generate image stacks at the exact same phase of the cardiac cycle. This results in a 4D dataset with data available for each position along the z-axis at every point of the R-R interval. Retrospective ECG-gating overcomes the limitations that are encountered during prospective ECG-triggering, thus, it is less susceptible to the heart rate changes during the scan. Retrospective gating also allows evaluation of cardiac function since volume data is acquired during the spiral CT scan. Coronary CT angiography with retrospective ECG-gating has been successfully used for the quantification of ventricular function [19], and proved to correlate well with echocardiographic and magnetic resonance assessment of the global ventricular function [20-22].

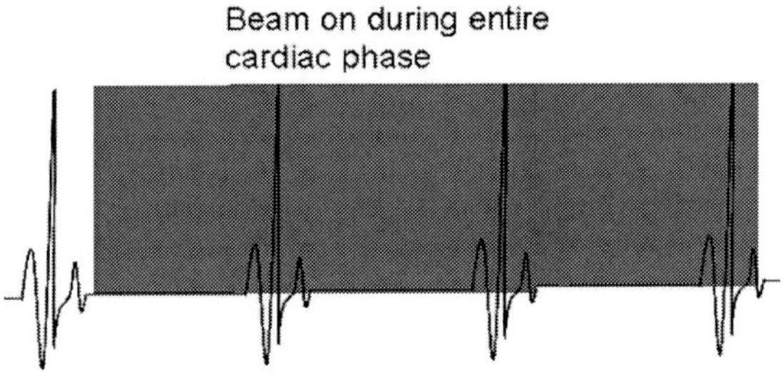

Figure 2.8. Conventional retrospectively ECG-gated coronary CT angiography. X-ray beam is turned on during the entire cardiac cycle without adjusting the tube current, allowing for acquisition of volume data.

However, the data is acquired at the expense of high radiation dose, since the table is advanced by less than one detector width during each gantry rotation; thus, the same anatomical area is exposed to X-ray radiation several times during consecutive rotations of the gantry, which results in higher radiation dose. The entire cardiac cycle is imaged as the patient moves continuously throughout the gantry. The radiation dose from retrospective ECG-gating ranges from 12 to 20 mSv, and could be as high as 40 mSv in female patients if no dose-saving strategies are applied [23, 24]. Different dose-saving strategies have been developed to minimize radiation dose, such as lower tube current during the systolic phase (tube current modulation), lower tube voltage, with resultant up to 40% dose reduction in coronary CT angiography [25-27].

2.2.3. Prospective ECG-triggering

Higher radiation dose associated with retrospectively ECG-gated coronary CT angiography has prompted the development of prospective ECG-triggering, as the latter involves scanning and reconstruction being performed during late diastolic phase.

Prospective ECG-triggering is a sequential scanning technique and it has long been used in conjunction with electron-beam CT and single-slice CT [28, 29]. In the sequential mode the CT scanner acquires the data of one slice during each gantry rotation, after which the table (and the patient) is advanced to the next plane position to acquire the next data of an adjacent slice, thus it is also called slice-by-slice acquisition or step-and-shoot mode (Figure 2.9). For coronary CT angiography with prospective ECG-triggering, a trigger signal is derived from the patient's ECG on the basis of a prospective estimation of the present R-R interval, and data is acquired in a certain predefined cardiac phase (in general the mid-to-end diastolic phase). Thereafter, the table moves to the next position, and the next scan is triggered to the next available R-wave. Prospectively ECG-triggered coronary CT angiography has been evaluated by clinical studies with promising results reported. A significant dose reduction has been achieved with up to 90% with use of prospective ECG-triggering when compared to retrospective ECG-gating [26, 30, 31]. This technique highly depends on a regular and low heart rate and is prone to motion artefacts as it tends to result in misregistration in the presence of arrhythmia. Moreover, there is a lack of inherent benefits of spiral CT, thus no volume data can be acquired with prospective ECG-triggering. Details about prospectively ECG-triggered coronary CT angiography will be discussed in Chapters 8-10.

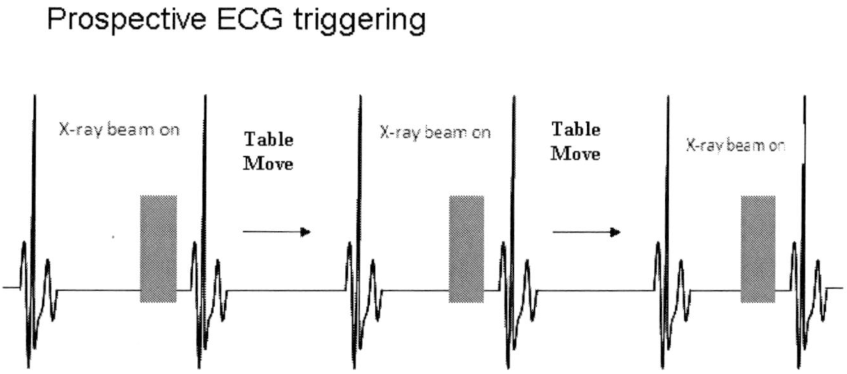

Figure 2.9. Prospectively ECG-triggered coronary CT angiography with X-ray beam on during a portion of cardiac cycle, while in the remaining cardiac phase, the X-ray beam is turned off.

2.3. Coronary CT Angiography-Postprocessing Techniques

The interpretation of coronary CT angiographic images performed with multislice CT scanners requires a number of postprocessing techniques and real-time interaction with the volumetric dataset that is generated. Image postprocessing is an essential part of spiral CT scans, especially CT angiography. This process involves generation and modification of a 3D volume data, which consists of a stack of individual 2D axial images. An ideal volume data of high spatial resolution should be isotropic in nature, i.e., each voxel has equal dimensions in all three dimensions (x, y and x-axes). This forms the basis for image display in advanced image postprocessing techniques as it can be performed arbitrarily at any oriented imaging planes to serve different visualization purposes. With the advent of multislice CT and the latest models such as 64- and more slice CT, isotropic volume data can be obtained for the majority of clinical examinations. The high spatial resolution of the reconstruted data allows for quantitative assessment of cardiac anatomy, ventricular function, ejection fraction and regional wall motion and wall thickening abnormalities [19-22]. This has improved the diagnostic quality of image postprocessing, in particular, forming a vital component for CT angiography [32-34].

The axial source images contain the basic information of a CT scan. The in-plane spatial resolution of original axial images determines the quality of reconstructed 2D and 3D images. For coronary CT angiography, in addition to 2D axial images, multiplanar reformation (MPR), maximum-intensity projection (MIP), volume rendering (VR) are the most commonly used tools for visualization and assessment of coronary arteries as well as the degree of coronary stenosis. Virtual intravascular endoscopy (VIE) is another 3D visualization tool which has been reported to provide useful information for assessment of coronary lumen and plaques [35].

In cardiac CT imaging, axial images are routinely viewed by scrolling through them up and down in the craniocaudal direction, which gives a quick overview of the relevant cardiac structures, including the normal coronary arteries and pathological changes such as coronary plaques. Figure 2.10 shows axial images acquired with a 64-slice CT scanner at different anatomical levels from a coronary CT angiography with demonstration of normal coronary artery branches.

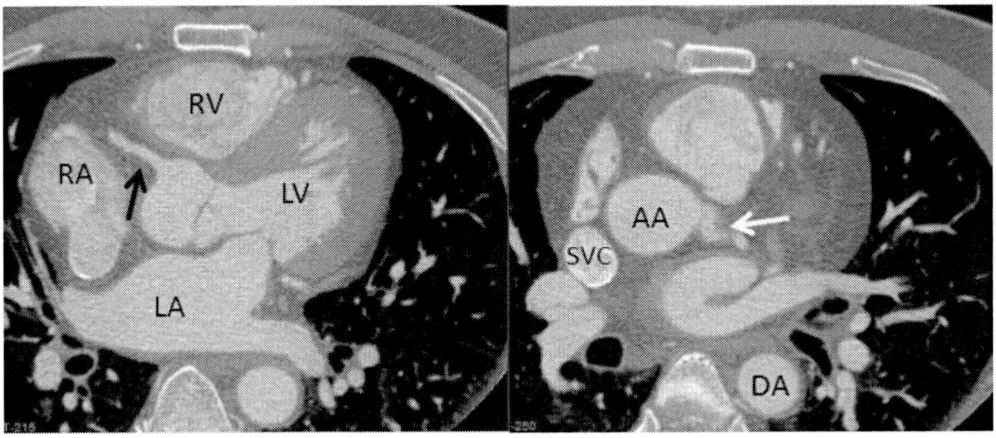

Figure 2.10. Axial images at different anatomical levels of a coronary CT angiography examination in a patient suspected of coronary artery disease. The images were acquired using a 64-slice CT scanner with 64 × 0.625 mm slices per rotation. Axial images include all of the information acquired in a CT scan and should be reviewed in any case, e.g., by scrolling through them. AA-ascending aorta, DA-descending aorta, SVC-superior vena cava, RA-right atrium, RV-right ventricle, LA-left atrium, LV-left ventricle. Black arrow indicates RCA, while the white arrow refers to LCA.

2.3.1. Multiplanar Reformation

MPR is the basic tool used to interpret coronary CT angiographic images. Simple examples of MPR are coronal and sagittal views which are widely used in general radiology but of limited use in cardiac imaging as coronary arteries demonstrate complex course and they do not follow a straight path along the cardiac muscle. Thus, a number of MPR images are required to demonstrate the entire course of coronary arteries, since not all of the coronary segments can be displayed in a single MPR view. Because of variations in the orientation of the heart in the thorax, it is generally recommended to evaluate cardiac structures along the cardiac planes for optimal evaluation of the cardiac anatomy.

2.3.2. Curved Planar Reformation

Since normal coronary arteries are often tortuous, accurate evaluation requires assessment of the entire vessel tree along its center line. CVR is the most useful visualization tool for cardiac CT as MPR views are generated along the curved planes instead of straight planes. Most cardiac workstations with cardiac analysis capabilities have software capable of automatically determining the center line of each coronary artery and display the entire length of the artery on a single CVR image (Figure 2.11) [5].

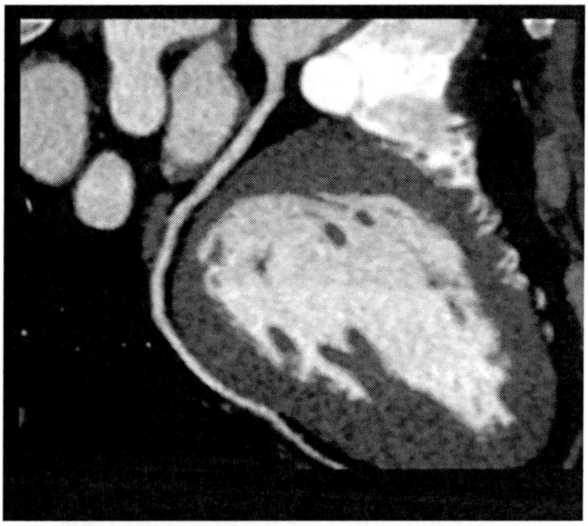

a

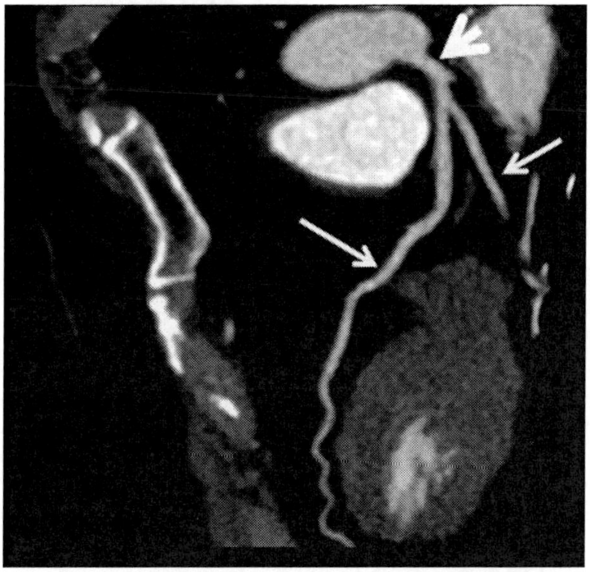

b

Figure 2.11. Curve planar reformatted (CVR) images show the normal RCA (A) and left main stem (arrowhead), LAD (long white arrow) and LCx (short white arrow).

2.3.3. Maximum-Intensity Projection

MIP is considered the most useful visualization tool in CT angiography as MIP images are similar to traditional angiograms, which display intraluminal opacity values, but provide angiographic-like images non-invasively. The principle of MIP visualization is the demonstration of only maximum CT number encountered in each ray. The differentiation between contrast-enhanced blood vessels and background is good, thus highest-attenuation structures typically contrast-enhanced arteries, bone and and calcification are preferentially depicted and displayed on MIP images (Figure 2.12). The limitation of MIP images is that they do not provide depth and spatial information regarding relationships to adjacent structures [36, 37]. Thin-slap MIPs are introduced to overcome this shortcoming. In particular, for diagnosis of the coronary arteries, planes in parallel to a line connecting RCA and LCx, and planes in parallel to a line along the LAD should be used to visualize the course of coronary arteries (Figure 2.13) [38].

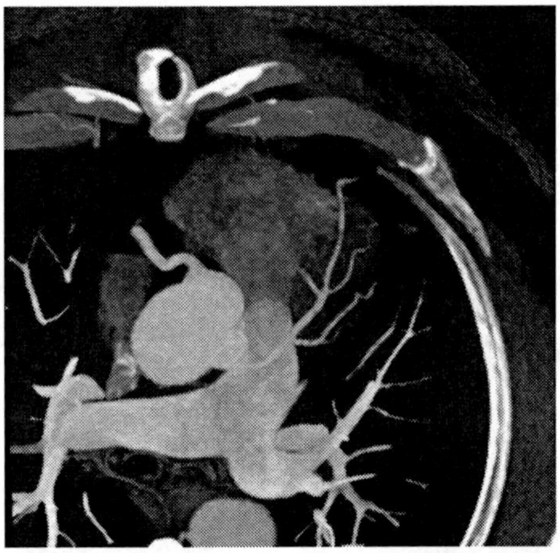

Figure 2.12. Axial MIP image shows the normal RCA.

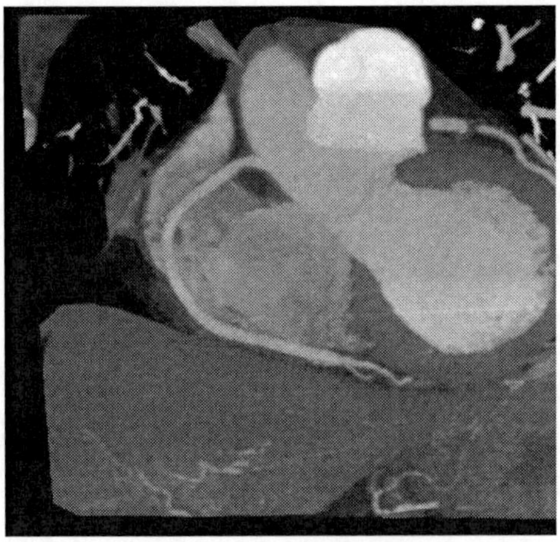

Figure 2.13. Thin-slab MIP image shows the normal RCA.

2.3.4. Volume Rendering

VR provides a 3D representation of the anatomical structures based on a volume dataset, since it utilizes all of the information contained in the data. A voxel-based intensity histogram is generated, and several parameters such as color, brightness and opacity are assigned to each voxel according to its CT attenuation value. Therefore, 3D relationship between different structures can be easily displayed and appreciated on VR, thereby producing an overall image of the heart, as shown in Figure 2.14. VR visualization facilitates surface evaluation of the heart and coronary arteries. VR requires extensive user interaction for accurate evaluation of complex anatomical structures. In most of the situation, segmentation of the overlapping structures is required, e.g. to remove the rib cage and pulmonary vessels for visualization of the heart and coronary arteries, thus, it could be a time-consuming task. Advanced cardiac software packages enable the heart to be automatically removed and VR display of the cardiac structures including coronary arteries becomes feasible without further segmentation.

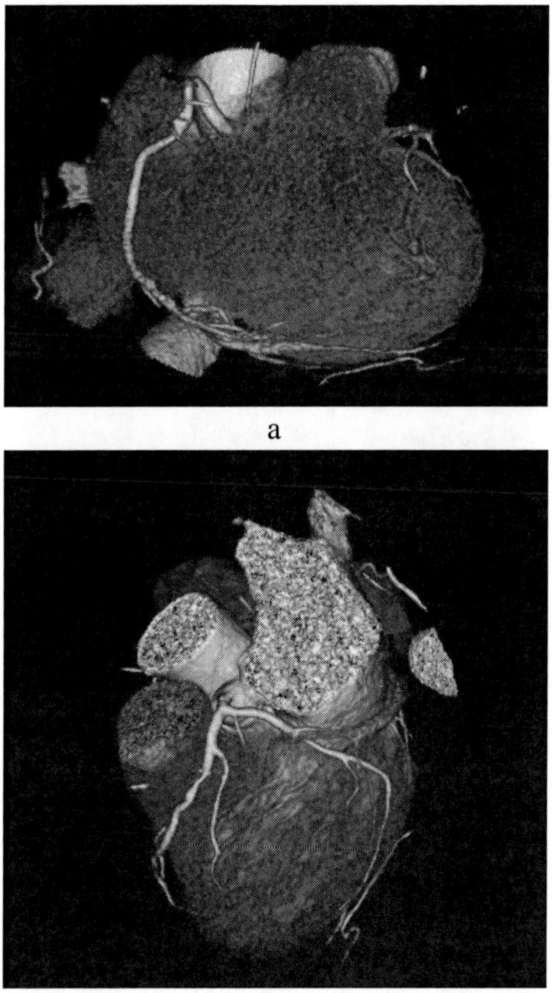

a

b

Figure 2.14. 3D volume rendering images clearly demonstrate the normal RCA (A), LAD and LCx (B).

2.3.5. Virtual Intravascular Endoscopy

Another 3D post-processing technique related to VR is VIE. VIE provides unique intravascular views of the blood vessels based on CT thresholding techniques [39, 40], thus, enabling visualization of coronary plaques and coronary lumen changes which cannot be obtained by traditional 2D or other 3D extraluminal views [35]. It offers additional information about the intraluminal appearance of coronary artery wall, coronary plaques and extent of coronary stenosis, although its clinical value in cardiac imaging remains to be proven. Figure 2.15 is an example of VIE visualization of normal coronary artery ostia, while Figure 2.16 shows an example of calcified plaques resulting in more than 50% of the coronary stenosis.

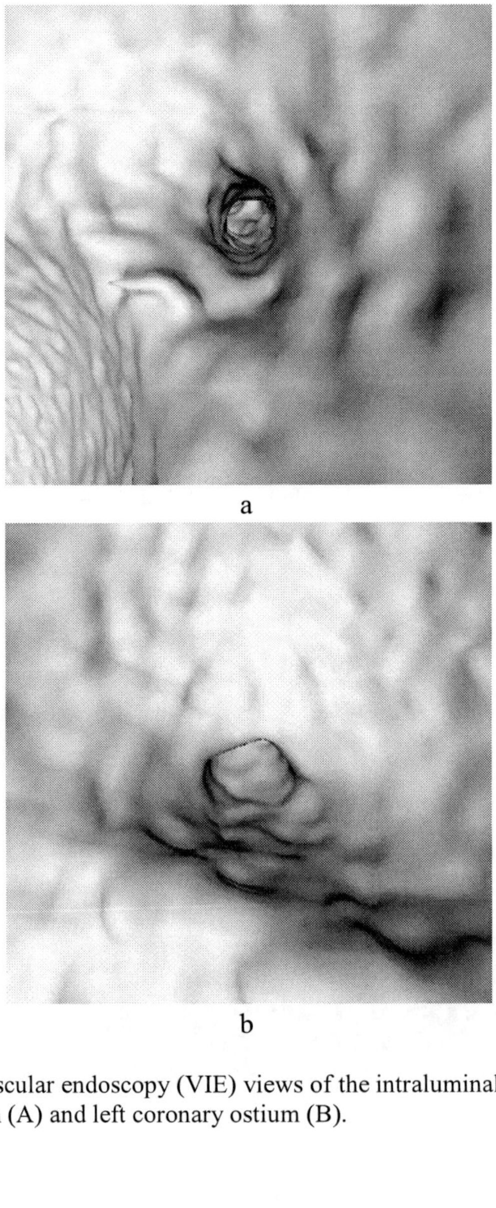

a

b

Figure 2.15. Virtual intravascular endoscopy (VIE) views of the intraluminal appearance of normal right coronary artery ostium (A) and left coronary ostium (B).

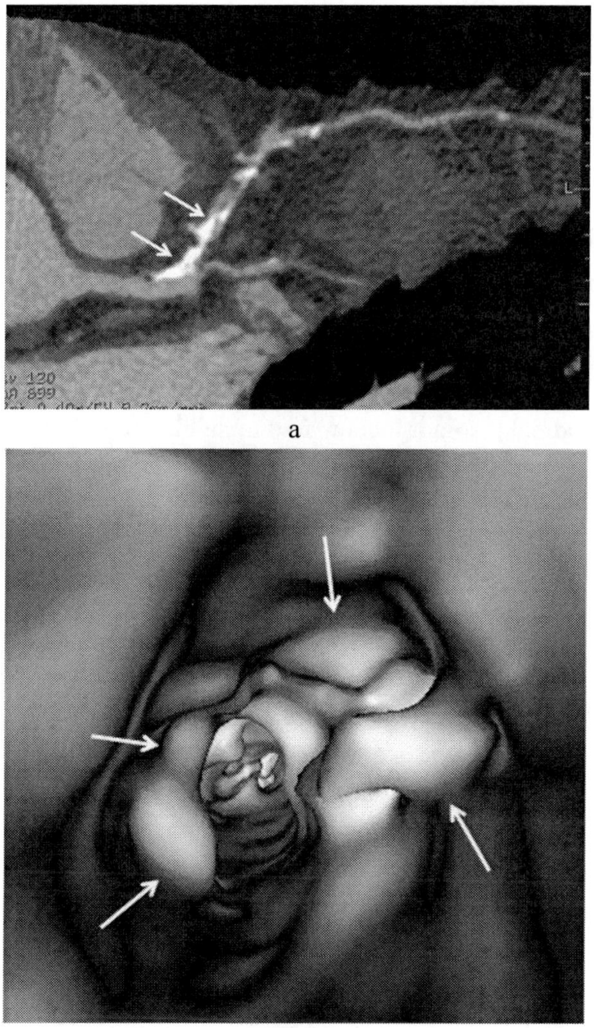

Figure 2.16. Calcified plaques are present in the left LAD (arrows in A), resulting in significant lumen stenosis. Corresponding VIE shows irregular coronary lumen changes (arrows in B) with more than 50% lumen stenosis.

2.3.6. Cine Imaging

Cine images are used for the purpose of demonstrating the motion and physiological features of cardiac structures such as the left ventricle and cardiac valves. The capabilities of the multislice CT scanners allow application of this technique, since data from the heart and coronary arteries are reconstructed at specific cardiac segments with least artefacts during cardiac cycle. Depending on the individual patient, the 40% series could represent end-systole, while the 90% series might correspond to end-diastole, with the remaining data points representing other phases of the cardiac cycle. Cine images are considered particularly useful for examining left ventricle wall motion and wall thickening and for assessing valve motion in multiple phases [4].

2.4. From 4-slice to 16-slice CT

The increased performance of multislice CT compared with single-slice CT significantly reduces the examination time for standard CT protocols, allows for immediate and comprehensive assessment of trauma and non-cooperative patients, and elimination of misregistration during breath-hold imaging. Also, the scan range can be extended by a factor of M (M=number of detector rows in multislice CT scanners) to allow coverage of longer anatomic regions within a shorter period, yet still produces high spatial resolution images [41, 42].

The most important clinical benefit for multislice CT lies in its ability to scan a given anatomic region within a given scan time with substantially reduced slice thickness, at M times increased longitudinal resolution compared to single-slice CT. The early generations of 4- and 16-slice CT scanners represented a technological revolution in cardiac imaging [43-45], although the diagnostic accuracy in terms of sensitivity was low for determining the degree of coronary artery disease (CAD). Specificity for exclusion of CAD (negative predictive value) was good and this generation of technology also proved useful for the evaluation of coronary anomalies and bypass graft patency. Improved spatial resolution with 16-slice CT plays an important role in the reliable detection and characterization of coronary plaques and cardiac wall changes (such as remodelling of the coronary wall due to atherosclerotic plaques). Longer anatomical coverage such as imaging of peripheral vascular system can be obtained with 16-slice CT with higher spatial (0.6 mm) and temporal resolution (165 ms) than early type of 4-slice CT scanners [46, 47]. However, the image quality is compromised in patients with high heart rate, or with stents or severely calcified arteries [48, 49].

2.5. 64-slice and Beyond

The introduction of 64-slice CT brought about a further leap in volume coverage speed. With gantry rotation times down to 330 ms for 64-slice CT, temporal resolution for ECG-gated cardiac imaging was again markedly improved. Improvement of image quality has also been reported in the visualization of all coronary artery branches with high sensitivity and specificity achieved [50-52]. In contrast to previous studies, high diagnostic accuracy has been obtained despite the presence of severely calcified coronary plaques. In patients with high heart rates, multisegment reconstruction algorithms were reported to provide diagnostic images by offering optimal temporal resolution, thus minimizing the occurrence of motion artefacts [53, 54].

Dual-source CT was designed to further improve temporal resolution to 83 ms, thus increasing image quality by reducing motion artefacts. Studies have shown a significant improvement with the use of coronary CT angiography in the assessment of patients with high heart rate when dual-source CT is used [15-18]. The development of wide area detector CT enables greater coverage per gantry rotation [55-57]. Expansion of multislice CT systems from a prototype 256-slice to a 320-slice system has allowed for acquisition of whole heart coverage in one gantry rotation. The 320-slice CT has one expanded 64-slice block along the z-axis and it can cover 16 cm (0.5 mm x 320 detectors) with an improved gantry rotation, resulting in excellent image quality and demonstration of the entire coronary arteries [58-60]. The 320-slice CT can scan the whole heart in less than 1 s, even in patients with an enlarged heart or in patients with atrial fibrillation, 320-slice CT produces sufficient image quality to diagnose coronary artery disease [56, 61]. More clinical data are being collected with regard to the diagnostic performance of 320-slice CT, and this will be discussed in Chapter 6.

Conclusion

Multislice CT has undergone rapid developments, which are reflected in high spatial and temporal resolution. Technical improvements in CT scanning have enabled acquisition of cardiac images within a very short time, but with sufficient image quality for diagnostic purpose. Successful performance of coronary CT angiography not only depends on careful selection of imaging protocols, but also relies on image postprocessing and visualization tools. In particular, multiplanar and 3D reconstruction tools have become a routine component of cardiac CT image analysis.

With 64- and more slice CT scanners becoming widely available, coronary CT angiography can be performed with high diagnostic accuracy. In some patients, coronary CT angiography is regarded as a reliable alternative to invasive coronary angiography, thus, serving as a screening technique for patients with suspected coronary artery disease. Further studies are needed to prove its clinical value as a routine imaging modality in cardiac imaging.

References

[1] Yang F, Minutello RM, Bhagan S, Sharma A, Wong SC. The impact of gender on vessel size in patients with angiographically normal coronary arteries. *J Interv Cardiol* 2006;19(4):340–344.

[2] Austen WG, Edwards JE, Frye RL, et al. A reporting system on patients evaluated for coronary artery disease. *Circulation* 1975;51(4 suppl):5– 40.

[3] Malouf JF, Edwards WD, Tajik AJ, Seward JB. Functional anatomy of the heart. In: Fuster V, Alexander RW, O'Rourke RA, Roberts R, King SB, Wellens HJJ, eds. *Hurst's the heart.* 11th ed. New York, NY: McGraw-Hill, 2005; 45–82.

[4] O'Brien JP, Srichai MB, Hecht EM, Kim DC, Jacobs JE. Anatomy of the Heart at multidetector CT: what the radiologist needs to know. *Radiographics* 2007; 27: 1569-1582.

[5] Hoffmann U, Pena AJ, Cury RC, et al. Cardiac CT in emergency department patients with acute chest pain. *RadioGraphics* 2006;26(4):963–980.

[6] Roberts WT, Bax JJ, Davies LC. Cardiac CT and CT coronary angiography: technology and application. *Heart* 2008; 94:781-792.

[7] Sun Z, Jiang W. Diagnostic value of multislice CT angiography in coronary artery disease: A meta-analysis. *Eur J Radiol* 2006; 60:279-286.

[8] Ohnesorge B, Becker C, Flohr T, Reiser MF. Multi-slice CT in cardiac imaging: technical principles, clinical application and future developments. Berlin, Germany: *Springer-Verlag,* 3–109, (2002).

[9] Sun Z, Lin CH, Davidson R, Dong C, Liao Y. Diagnostic value of 64-slice CT angiography in coronary artery disease: A systematic review. *Eur J Radiol* 2008; 67:78-84.

[10] Flohr T, Ohnesorge B. Heart rate adaptive optimization of spatial and temporal resolution for electrocardiogram-gated multislice spiral CT of the heart. *J Comput Assist Tomogr* 2001; 25:907– 923.

[11] De Roos A, Kroft LJ, Bax JJ, Lamb HJ, Geleijns J. Cardiac applications of multislice computed tomography. *Br J Radiol* 2006; 79:9-16.

[12] Desjardins B, Kazerooni EA. ECG-Gated Cardiac CT. *AJR Am J Roentgenol* 2004;182:993–1010.

[13] Achenbach S, Ropers D, Holle J, Muschiol G, Daniel WG, Moshage W. In-plane coronary arterial motion velocity: measurement with electron-beam CT. *Radiology* 2000; 216:457–463.

[14] Kuetter A, Beck T, Drosch T, et al. Image quality and diagnostic accuracy of non-invasive coronary imaging with 16 detector slice spiral computed tomography with 188 ms temporal resolution. *Heart* 2005; 91: 938-941.

[15] Flohr TG, McCollough CH, Bruder H, et al. First performance evaluation of a dual source CT (DSCT) system. *Eur Radiol* 2006; 16:256-268.

[16] Brodoefel H, Burgstahler C, Tsiflikas I, et al. Dual-Source CT: Effect of heart rate, heart rate variability, and calcification on image quality and diagnostic accuracy. *Radiology* 2008; 247:346-355.

[17] Johnson T, Nikolaou K, Busch S, et al. Diagnostic accuracy of dual-source computed tomography in the diagnosis of coronary artery disease. *Invest Radiol* 2007; 42: 484-491.

[18] Leber AW, Johnson T, Becker A, et al. Diagnostic accuracy of dual-source multi-slice CT coronary angiography in patients with an intermediate pretest likelihood for coronary artery disease. *Eur Heart J* 2007; 28:2354-2360.

[19] Raman SV, Shah M, McCarthy B, et al. Multidetector row cardiac computed tomography accurately quantifies right and left ventricular size and function compared with cardiac magnetic resonance. *Am Heart J* 2006 ; 151 : 736-744.

[20] Schlosser T, Pagonidis K, Herborn CU, et al. Assessment of left ventricular parameter using 16-MDCT and new software for endocardial and epicardial border delineation. *AJR Am J Roentgenol* 2005 ; 184 : 765-773.

[21] Lessick J, Mutlak D, Rispler S, et al. Comparison of multidetector computed tomography versus echocardiography for assessing regional left ventricular function. *Am J Cardiol* 2005; 96: 1011-1015.

[22] Mahnken AH, Muhlenbruch G, Gunther RW, et al. Cardiac CT: coronary arteries and beyond. *Eur Radiol* 2007; 17: 994-1008.

[23] Sabarudin A, Sun Z, Ng KH. A systematic review of radiation dose associated with different generations of multislice CT coronary angiography. *J Med Imaging Radiat Oncol* 2012; 56: 5-17.

[24] Husmann L, Valenta I, Gaemperli O, et al. Feasibility of low-dose coronary CT angiography: first experience with prospective ECG-gating. *Eur Heart J* 2008; 29: 191-197.

[25] Hassan A, Nazir SA, Alkadhi H. Technica challenges of coronary CT angiography : today and tomorrow. *Eur J Radiol* 2011 ; 79 : 161-171.

[26] Sun Z, Ng KH. Multislice CT angiography in cardiac imaging: Part III: Radiation risk and dose reduction. *Singapore Med J* 2010; 51: 374-380.

[27] Sun Z, Choo, Ng KH. Coronary CT angiography: current status and continuing challenges. *Br J Radiol* 2012; 85: 495-510.

[28] Schoepf UJ, Becker CR, Bruening RD, et al. Electrocardiographically gated thinsection CT of the lung. *Radiology* 1999; 212:649–654.

[29] Becker CR, Jakobs TF, Aydemir S, et al. Helical and single-slice conventional CT versus electron beam CT for the quantification of coronary artery calcification. *AJR Am J Roentgenol* 2000; 174:543–547.

[30] Sun Z. Multislice CT angiography in cardiac imaging: prospective ECG-gating or retrospective ECG-gating? *Biomed Imaging Intervent J* 2010; 6(1) e4.

[31] Sun Z, Ng KH. Diagnostic value of coronary CT angiography with prospective ECG-gating in the diagnosis of coronary artery disease: A systematic review and meta-analysis. *Int J Cardiovasc Imaging* 2012; 28: 2109-2119..

[32] Addis KA, Hopper KD, Iyriboz TA, et al. CT angiography: in vitro comparison of five reconstruction methods. *AJR Am J Roentgenol* 2001; 177:1171–1176.

[33] Prokop M, Shin HO, Schanz A, Schaefer-Prokop CM. Use of maximum intensity projections in CT angiography: a basic review. *Radiographics* 1997; 17:433–51.

[34] Rankin CS. CT angiography (Review). *Eur Radiol* 1999; 9:297–310.

[35] Sun Z, Dimpudus FJ, Nugroho J, Adipranoto JD. CT virtual intravascular endoscopy assessment of coronary artery plaques: A preliminary study. *Eur J Radiol* 2010; 75: e112-e119.

[36] Gruden JF. Thoracic CT performance and interpretation in the multi-detector era. *J Thorac Imaging* 2005;20(4):253–264.

[37] Cody DD. AAPM/RSNA physics tutorial for residents: topics in CT—image processing in CT. *RadioGraphics* 2002;22(5):1255–1268.

[38] Ohnesorge B, Flohr T, Becker , Knez A, Reiser M. Multi-slice and dual-source CT in cardiac imaging: principles, protocols, indications, outlook, 2nd ed. Berlin, Germany: *Springer-Verlag,* 151-176, (2007).

[39] Sun Z, Winder RJ, Kelly BE, Ellis PK, Kennedy PT, Hirst DG. Diagnostic value of CT virtual intravascular endoscopy in aortic stent grafting. *J Endovasc Ther* 2004; 11(1):13-25.

[40] Sun Z, Winder RJ, Kelly BE, Ellis PK, Hirst DG. CT virtual intravascular endoscopy of abdominal aortic aneurysms treated with suprarenal endovascular stent grafting. *Abdom Imaging* 2003; 28(4):580-587.

[41] Knez A, Becker C, Leber A, Ohnesorge B, Reiser M, Haberl R. Noninvasive assessment of coronary artery stenoses with multidetector helical computed tomography. *Circulation* 2000; 101: e221-e222.

[42] Prokop M. General principles of MDCT. *Eur J Radiol* 2003; 45:S4-S10.

[43] Nieman K, Oudkerk M, Rensing BJ, et al. Coronary angiography with multi-slice computed tomography. *Lancet* 2001; 357: 599-603.

[44] Kuettner A, Trabold T, Schroeder S, et al. Noninvasive detection of coronary artery lesions using 16-detector row multislice spiral computed tomography technology: initial clinical results. *J Am Coll Cardiol* 2004; 44: 1230-7.

[45] Achenbach S, Giesler T, Ropers D, et al. Detection of coronary artery stenoses by contrast-enhanced, retrospectively electrocardiographically-gated multislice computed tomography. *Circulation* 2001; 103: 2535-2538.

[46] Nieman K, Cademartiri F, Lemos PA, Raaijmakers R, Pattynama PM, de Feyter PJ. Reliable noninvasive coronary angiography with fast submillimeter multislice spiral computed tomography. *Circulation* 2002; 106:2051-2054.

[47] Achenbach S, Ropers D, Pohle FK, D. et al. Detection of coronary artery stenoses using multi-detector CT with 16 x 0.75 collimation and 375 ms rotation. *Eur Heart J* 2005; 26:1978-1986.

[48] Achenbach S. Detection of coronary stenoses by multidetector computed tomography: it is all about resolution. *J Am Coll Cardiol* 2004; 43:840-841.

[49] Flohr TG, Schoepf UJ, Kuettner A, et al. Advances in cardiac imaging with 16-section CT systems. *Acad Radiol* 2003; 10:386-401.

[50] Pugliese F, Mollet NR, Runza G, et al. Diagnostic accuracy of non-invasive 64-slice CT coronary angiography in patients with stable angina pectoris. *Eur Radiol,* 2006;16:575-582.

[51] Ong TK, Chin SP, Liew CK, et al. Accuracy of 64-row multidetector computed tomography in detecting coronary artery disease in 134 symptomatic patients: influence of calcification. *Am Heart J* 2006; 151:1323.e1–6.

[52] Raff GL, Gallagher MJ, O'Neill WW, Goldstein JA. Diagnostic accuracy of non-invasive coronary angiography using 64-slice spiral computed tomography. *J Am Coll Cardiol* 2005, 46: 552-557.

[53] Wintersperger BJ, Nikolaou K, von Ziegler F, et al. Image quality, motion artifacts, and reconstruction timing of 64-slice coronary computed tomography angiography with 0.33-second rotation speed. *Invest Radiol* 2006;41: 436–442.

[54] Herzog C, Nguyen SA, Savino G, et al. Does two-segment image reconstruction at 64-section CT coronary angiography improve image quality and diagnostic accuracy? *Radiology* 244(1):121–129.

[55] Chao SP, Law WY, Kuo CJ, Hung HF, Cheng JJ, Lo HM, Shyu KG. The diagnostic accuracy of 256-row computed tomographic angiography compared with invasive coronary angiography in patients with suspected coronary artery disease. *Eur Heart J* 2010; 31: 1916-1923.

[56] Rybicki F, Otero H, Steigner M, et al. Initial evaluation of coronary images from 320-detector row computed tomography. *Int J Cardiovasc Imaging* 2008; 24: 535-546.

[57] Dewey M, Deissenrieder ZF, Laule M, et al. Noninvasive coronary angiography by 320-row computed tomography with lower radiation exposure and maintained diagnostic accuracy: comparison of results with cardiac catheterization in a head-to-head pilot investigation. *Circulation* 2009;120: 867-875.

[58] Hoe J, Toh KH. First experience with 320-row multidetector CT coronary angiography scanning with prospective electrocardiogram gating to reduce radiation dose. *J Cardiovasc Comput Tomogr* 2009;3:257-261.

[59] De Graaf FR, Schuijf JD, van Velzen JE, et al. Diagnostic accuracy of 320-row multidetector computed tomography coronary angiography in the non-invasive evaluation of significant coronary artery disease. *Eur Heart J* 2010; 31: 1908-1915.

[60] Nasis A, Leung MC, Antonis PR, et al. Diagnostic accuracy of noninvasive coronary angiography with 320-detector row computed tomography. *Am J Cardiol* 2010; 106: 1429-1435.

[61] Pasricha SS, Nandurkar D, Seneviratne SK, et al. Image quality of coronary 320-MDCT in patients with atrial fibrillation: initial experience. *AJR Am J Roentgenol* 2009; 193: 1514-1521.

Chapter 3

Coronary CT Angiography: Radiation Dose Measurements and Dose Reduction Strategies

Abstract

This chapter provides an overview of the radiation dose measurements that are commonly used in coronary CT angiography, and the strategies that are recently undertaken and recommended to reduce radiation dose from coronary CT angiography. It is of paramount importance to be aware of the fact that CT is a high-dose imaging modality, and the necessity to minimize radiation dose when performing coronary CT angiography. Significant progress has been achieved over the last few years with regard to dose reduction in coronary CT angiography, with dose level equal to or lower than that acquired from invasive coronary angiography.

Keywords: Coronary CT angiography, CT dosimetry, dose reduction, radiation dose

3.1. Introduction

Radiation dose is becoming a major issue for coronary CT angiography, since 64- or more-slice CT shows improved and promising results in the diagnosis of coronary artery disease (CAD) [1-4]. It is estimated that in daily practice, median doses of coronary CT angiography differ significantly between study sites and CT systems, with up to 6-fold differences in dose measurement indicating the large variability in coronary CT angiography protocols [5]. Cardiac patients may also be exposed to other sources of medical radiation (including from nuclear medicine and invasive coronary angiography examinations). With repeated examinations and the cumulated radiation dose, radiation exposure has become a definite risk to patients. Given the fact that CT is a high-dose imaging modality, it is essential to minimize the radiation dose associated with coronary CT angiographic examinations.

Many clinicians may still be unfamiliar with the magnitude of radiation exposure arising from coronary CT angiography in daily practice and with factors that contribute to the radiation dose. Therefore, the benefit of the using coronary CT angiography in the diagnostic workup and patient management must be weighed against the potential risks related to radiation exposure. Recently, tremendous progress has been made to lower radiation dose for coronary CT angiography. It is obvious that the strategies to lower the overall radiation exposure to the population must be twofold: first, the radiation dose of the individual CT study should be lowered to a level that is as low as reasonably achievable (ALARA); and second, the total number of coronary CT angiography studies must be determined by adhering to strict guidelines and recommendations [6]. Strategies to reduce radiation exposure in coronary CT angiography have been developed and include anatomy-based tube current modulation, electrocardiography (ECG)-based tube current modulation, reduced X-ray tube voltage, high pitch value and synchronization to the cardiac cycle-prospectively triggered axial acquisition [7-10]. This chapter will provide an overview of the parameters for CT dose measurements, and the strategies currently available to address radiation dose reduction associated with coronary CT angiography.

3.2. CT Dosimetry Measurements

Patient exposure in CT is different from in conventional X-ray examinations, as the X-ray tube rotates around the patient from all angle producing thin slices of the irradiated body region during CT image acquisition. Thus, dose calculation in CT is more complicated and requires the introduction of special dosimetric quantities such as CT Dose Index (CTDI) for a single slice and the Dose Length Product (DLP) for a complete examination [11]. With introduction of multislice CT scanners, volumetric CTDI (CTDIvol) was introduced in order to determine the dose in one gantry rotation.

3.2.1. CT Dose Index

The fundamental radiation dose parameter in CT is the CTDI. The CTDI is usually measured with a pencil ionization chamber with an active length of 100 mm both in free air at the center of rotation and within cylindrical phantoms of 16 and 32 cm in diameter, simulating the head and body of a patient, respectively. CTDI $_{100}$ is a measured parameter of radiation exposure which is more convenient than the CTDI and it is regarded as the measurement of choice performed by medical physicists in the clinical setting [12]. It is obtained with an ionization chamber that integrates the radiation exposure of a single axial scan over a length of 100 mm [13]. The weighted CTDI (CTDIw) is the weighted average of the CTDI $_{100}$ measurements at the center and the peripheral locations of the phantom. This parameter reflects the average absorbed dose over the two-dimensions (x and y dimensions) of the average radiation dose to a cross-section of a patient's body.

The volume CTDI (CTDIvol) is a relatively new radiation dose parameter agreed on by the International Electrotechnical Commission [14]. The CTDIvol is introduced to determine the radiation dose in one tube rotation in multislice CT scanners and allows for variations in exposure in the z direction. It is different from CTDIw as the former averages radiation dose over three-dimensions (x, y, and z directions) (CTDIw represents the average exposure in the x-y plane only) [12]. CTDIvol is the weighted CTDI divided by the pitch, or CTDIvol=

CTDIw /pitch. The CTDIvol is now the preferred radiation dose parameter in CT dosimetry. Current multislice CT scanners can display the CTDIvol values on the operator's console. This allows the clinician to directly compare the radiation doses that patients receive from different imaging protocols. Similar to the CTDIw, the CTDIvol is expressed in milligray (mGy).

3.2.2. Dose-Length Product

The DLP is used to calculate the dose for a series of slices and is an indicator of the integrated radiation dose of an entire CT examination [12]. The DLP is an approximation of the total energy a patient absorbs from the scan. It incorporates the number of scans and the scan width, e, g. the total scan length, while in contrast CTDIw and CTDIvol represent the radiation dose of an individual slice or scan. Therefore, DLP increases with an increase in total scan length or variables that affect the CTDIw (e.g. tube voltage or tube current) or the CTDIvol (e.g. pitch). Because scan length is expressed in centimeters, the SI unit for DLP is mGycm. Similar to CTDIvol, DLP is also available on the operator's console.

3.2.3. Effective Dose

The most important parameter in CT imaging is the effective dose, which is a dose parameter that reflects the risk of a non-uniform exposure in terms of a whole body exposure. It is valuable in assessing and comparing the potential biological risk of a specific examination [15]. The SI unit of measuring effective dose is the sievert (Sv) or millisievert (mSv). The effective dose is calculated from information about dose to individual organs and the relative radiation risk assigned to each organ [15].

The calculation of the effective dose in the current literature is based on a method proposed by the European Working Group for Guidelines on Quality Criteria in CT [16], deriving radiation dose estimates from the product of the DLP and an organ weighting factor for the chest as the investigated anatomic region ($k = 0.014$ or 0.017 mSv mGy^{-1} cm^{-1}) averaged between male and female models from Monte Carlo simulations [17]. Effective dose allows comparison across the different types of CT studies and between CT and other imaging test, facilitating comparison of CT to the most common radiology studies. The International Commission on Radiological Protection (ICRP) emphasizes that effective dose is intended for use as a protection quantity on the basis of reference values and therefore should not be used for epidemiological evaluations, nor should it be used for any specific investigations of human exposure [11].

The use of effective dose for assessing the exposure to patients undergoing coronary CT angiography has several limitations. An effective dose allows comparison of the use of similar technologies and procedures in different hospitals and countries as well as from use of different technologies for the same medical examinations. However, an effective dose does not tell the complete story with regard to the potential effects of ionizing radiation, as specific organs and tissues are known to be more radiosensitive than others.

A recent systematic review of coronary CT angiography with use of prospective ECG-triggering versus retrospective gating shows that in characterizing a cardiac CT study, DLP is a more objective physics metric than effective dose [18]. The variability of DLP between different study sites observed in this review was striking, as the DLP reported in the studies ranged from 129 mGy cm to 337 mGy cm. Median DLP at the highest dose sites was more than 3 times that at the lowest dose sites. Thus, coronary CT angiography may be associated with significantly higher or lower dose than invasive coronary angiography, depending on how CT angiography is performed at a study site. The DLP represents most closely the radiation dose received by an individual patient and may be used to set reference values for a given type of CT examination to help ensure patient doses at CT are as low as reasonably achievable. It is recommended that DLP should be recorded for each study and serve as the cornerstone of quality assurance efforts [19].

3.3. Strategies for Dose Reduction

Selection of scanning parameters for coronary CT angiography is a complex task and depends to a large extent on the anatomical region to be scanned, the size and the pathology of the patient. The chosen parameters should result in adequate image quality for clinical diagnosis. The main concern in determining exposure parameters is image noise and its effect on image quality. Some common parameters that affect the image quality and radiation dose of coronary CT angiography are discussed in the following sections.

3.3.1. Anatomy-Based Tube Current Modulation

Automatic tube current modulation technique is used to maintain diagnostic images while reducing radiation exposure on the basis of patient geometry (anatomy-adapted tube current modulation). It is regarded as an effective dose-saving algorithm, as the tube current is adjusted according to the patient's size, anatomic shape or both (e.g. the tube current is increased for obese patients or high attenuation projections such as lateral projections and decreased for small patients or low attenuation projections to generate a diagnostic image quality at the lowest dose).

Adjustment of the tube current can be performed in three-dimensional directions, including x, y (angular modulation), and z-axes (longitudinal modulation). Hence, automatic tube current modulation is analogous to the automatic exposure control or photograph-timing techniques used on conventional radiography [20].

It has been reported that automatic tube current modulation was an effective method of reducing radiation dose by 20-60%, depending on the anatomic regions and patient's habitus [21, 22].

However, automatic tube current modulation is expected to play a limited role in dose reduction in coronary CT angiography because of the relatively smaller angular or z-axis fluctuation of attenuation at the heart level [23]. Advanced tube current modulation schemes such as organ-based tube current modulation are being developed to reduce radiation dose to superficial radiation-sensitive tissues such as the breast without affecting image noise [24].

3.3.2. ECG-Controlled Tube Current Modulation

One of the effective approaches for radiation dose reduction in coronary CT angiography is achieved with ECG-controlled tube current modulation. Most of the coronary CT angiography scans are performed using retrospectively ECG-gated technique, which indicates that the volume data are acquired during the entire cardiac cycle within a single breath-hold helical scan. However, image reconstruction of the data only takes place in a specific phase of the cardiac cycle (end systole or mid diastole). This implies that tube current can be adjusted in different cardiac phases so that high-quality diagnostic images of coronary arteries during the reconstruction window, and low-quality, higher noise images of the cardiac chamber and cardiac valves during the rest of cardiac cycle can be acquired. This algorithm restricts the prescribed tube current to a pre-defined time window during the diastolic phase and decreases tube current in the systolic phase of the cardiac cycle [6], thus achieving significant dose reduction with this method. With this technique, the tube current outside the diastole is lowered to 25% of the nominal value, thus, the effective dose can be significantly lowered, with a drop of effective dose to around 10 mSv [5, 6, 25].

ECG-controlled tube current modulation has been reported to reduce radiation dose by 30-50% [26, 27]. ECG-controlled tube current modulation was more effective in patients with low and regular heart rates during the CT scan, however, the full tube current window was applied in patients with high or irregular/variable heart rates, which leads to the significant effect of heart rate and rhythm on radiation dose [28]. Yang et al in their recent study performed with 256-slice CT coronary angiography reported the feasibility of using heart rate-dependent ECG-pulsed tube current modulation [29]. Radiation dose can be considerably reduced, especially in patients with heart rate < 72 beats per minute (bpm) or >85 bpm, according to this study. Latest CT models such as 256- and 320-slice CT could address the limitation of fast or variable heart rates, although more evidence is needed.

3.3.3. Lower Tube Voltage

Another effective method currently undertaken in clinical practice to reduce radiation dose is to lower the tube voltage (kV). Lowering the tube voltage represents an important radiation dose reduction approach because the radiation dose varies with the square of the kV. Lowering the tube voltage has another additional advantage of the higher attenuation levels for iodinated contrast medium due to a greater photoelectric effect and decreased Compton scattering [30].

Modern CT scanners include tube voltages of 120 or 140 kV, reflecting the settings most often resulting in adequate image quality. However, cardiac CT acquisition with 100 kV, or even lower, is possible and has been suggested as an effective means to reduce radiation dose in cardiac CT imaging. It has been shown that decreasing the X-ray tube voltage from 120 to 80 kV resulted in a 70% reduction in radiation exposure for a constant tube current using 16- and 64-slice CT, with increased image noise and unchanged contrast-to-noise ratio [9, 31]. Studies utilising dual-source CT compared a 100 kV protocol to the routine 120 kV for cardiac CT, and demonstrated a 25–54% reduction in radiation dose, with an estimated effective dose as low as 4.4 mSv [30, 32,33].

In the PROTECTION 1 study reducing the tube voltage to 100 kV resulted in a 53% reduction in the median radiation dose for coronary CT angiography when compared to the conventional 120 kV scan protocol [34]. Diagnostic image quality was not affected, despite the increase of image noise. It must be noted that lowering of the tube voltage should be done according to the body mass index (BMI) of the patient. Lowering the tube voltage from 120 to 100 kV is appropriate when the patient's BMI is <25 kg/m^2. Reduction of the tube voltage to 80 kV should only be considered in children and slim young adults with a BMI <20 kg/m^2.

3.3.4. ECG-Gated High-Pitch Protocol

For the assessment of coronary arteries, coronary CT angiography is most commonly performed with spiral acquisition with low pitch values (0.2 to 0.4) and retrospective ECG-gating, which is associated with substantial oversampling. This indicates that the same level is irradiated during several consecutive rotations of the X-ray gantry, resulting in high radiation dose [35].

A dual-source CT scanner has greater temporal resolution, so the pitch may vary automatically with the heart rate. With dual-source scanners, the pitch can be increased at higher heart rates, resulting in a faster table speed and a corresponding reduction in radiation exposure. Pitch ranging from 0.25 at lower heart rates to 0.5 at high heart rates was possible with use of dual-source CT, resulting in coverage of the entire heart volume within 5-10 s, thus, dose was decreased accordingly from the pitch adaptation based on heart rates [36, 37].

The amount of radiation reduction is dependent on the patient's heart rate. Ketelsen et al [38] in their study based on a Randon phantom showed a significant reduction of radiation dose with increased heart rate because of the effect of increased pitch values resulting in less overlapping and reduced radiation dose. They concluded that a dose reduction of 31.9% for coronary CT angiography and 29.6% for calcium scoring with dual-source CT scans was achieved at a heart rate of 100 bpm (pitch 0.5) when compared to the scans performed at a heart rate of 40 bpm (pitch 0.2). An increased heart rate tends to degrade image quality in cardiac CT imaging with single-source CT, thus, an aggressive approach such as administration of beta-blockers prior to CT scanning is commonly used to lower the patient's heart rate [39]. The improved temporal resolution of dual-source CT results in a robust image quality within a wide range of heart rates; thus provides the opportunity to image patients with higher heart rates without requiring pre-examination use of beta-blockers [38-41].

One of the most recent developments in dose-saving strategies for coronary CT angiography is the ECG-triggered high-pitch protocol. With this protocol, data is acquired in a spiral model while the table moves with a high pitch of up to 3.4, equalling a table feed of 46 cm/s. When using the high-pitch protocol, the entire heart can be scanned within one single cardiac cycle, usually during diastole. Studies using dual-source CT in coronary CT angiography shows the feasibility of high-pitch spiral acquisition with prospective ECG-triggering [42-47]. Diagnostic image quality with very low radiation dose (0.78-2.1 mSv) was achieved in the majority of patients by prospectively ECG-triggered high-pitch coronary CT angiography (pitch 3.2-3.4). Effective radiation dose can be even lowered to less than 1 mSv with prospective ECG-triggering technique [42, 43, 47].

3.3.5. Prospective ECG-Triggering

Another significant leap in radiation dose reduction of coronary CT angiography is the introduction of prospective ECG-triggering, or the step-and-shoot mode. Prospective ECG-triggering is characterized by turning on the X-ray tube only at a predefined time point of the cardiac cycle, usually in diastole, while keeping the patient table stationary, and moving to the next location for another scan that is initiated by the subsequent cardiac cycle. In prospective triggering, radiation is only administered at predefined time points of the cardiac cycle, instead of the entire cardiac cycle as observed in the retrospectively-gated helical model, thus, a significant dose reduction is achieved with use of this scanning protocol, which ranges from 1 to 4 mSv, according to some early reports [48-51]. Coronary CT angiography performed with prospective ECG-triggering has been reported to have similar or improved image quality but up to 90% lower patient dose when compared with use of retrospectively ECG-gated protocol [52-54].

According to a number of systematic review and meta-analysis reports, the mean effective radiation dose for prospectively ECG-triggered coronary CT angiography in patients with a low and regular heart rate ranges from 2.7 mSv to 4.5 mSv [18, 55, 56], which is significantly lower than that for retrospectively ECG-gated coronary CT angiography. Further reduction of radiation dose can be achieved in prospectively ECG-triggered coronary CT angiography with use of lower kV values and high-pitch mode. A reduction of effective dose by up to 55% has been reported in prospective ECG-triggering with application of 80 and 100 kV without compromising image quality [18, 55]. Therefore, a combination of prospective ECG-triggering with a low kV protocol should be recommended in patients with BMI less than 25 kg/m^2, since changing tube voltage needs to be correlated with the patient's BMI.

Generally, prospectively ECG-triggered coronary CT angiography is only feasible in patients with a low and regular heart rate, since this scanning protocol requires the use of strict exclusion criteria, thus, patients with higher heart rates are normally excluded. With latest CT models, such as 320-slice CT, high diagnostic accuracy of coronary CT angiography has been achieved with use of prospective triggering in patients with high or irregular heart rates [57, 58], with radiation dose similar to that from invasive coronary angiography. 320-slice CT has the potential to broaden the application of coronary CT angiography to more patients such as patients with atrial fibrillation, although further studies, particularly, studies based on multi-center trials should be conducted to confirm its clinical value.

3.3.6. Iterative Reconstructions

The iterative reconstruction is an image reconstruction algorithm which is known for the potential to reduce image noise, artefacts and dose. It has been used extensively in emission tomographic modalities such as single photon emission computed tomography and positron emission tomography. In CT, however, this method is not currently in use on most of the medical scanners mainly due to its much computationally demanding and time-consuming when compared to the filtered back projection methods which are currently available on all commercial CT scanners. The benefit of iterative reconstruction on clinical application is that the low noise feature of iterative reconstruction can be applied to those examinations requiring high quality of images, but with a much lower dose [21].

More recently, different iterative image reconstruction methods for reducing radiation dose without compromising image quality have been developed by all major CT manufacturers: adaptive statistical iterative reconstruction (ASIR) and model based iterative reconstruction (MBIR) (GE Healthcare), iterative reconstruction in image space (IRIS) (Siemens Medical Solutions), adaptive iterative dose reduction (AIDR) (Toshiba Medical Systems) and iDose (Philips Healthcare) [59]. Clinical evaluation has shown up to 60% dose reduction compared to standard filtered back projection while maintaining diagnostic images [60, 61]. Coronary CT angiography incorporating iterative reconstruction resulted in a significant reduction in the effective dose.

Conclusion

It is important to be aware of the amount of radiation dose associated with coronary CT angiography and to realize that a careful selection of CT scanning protocols is required to keep the radiation exposure ALARA. This chapter demonstrates the radiation dose measurements in cardiac CT imaging and highlights the various strategies that have been undertaken recently to reduce the radiation exposure to patients undergoing coronary CT angiography. The radiation dose of coronary CT angiography can be reduced significantly with use of these dose-saving strategies. With successful implementation of these techniques, the effective dose of coronary CT angiography can be reduced to as low as 1 mSv in selected patients. It is important to note that the current effective doses from coronary CT angiography are at the level or even lower than those reported for the invasive coronary angiography. Therefore, tremendous progress has been achieved in radiation dose reduction in coronary CT angiography. Further research should focus on developing patient-based and technology-based methods to achieve the aim of reducing radiation dose while maintaining diagnostic image quality. Another important issue is to make sure that all these low-dose protocols for coronary CT angiography are widely used by the large radiological community performing cardiac imaging.

References

[1] Raff GL, Gallagher MJ, O'Neill WW, et al. Diagnostic accuracy of non-invasive coronary angiography using 64-slice spiral computed tomography. *J Am Coll Cardiol* 2005, 46:552-557.

[2] Chao SP, Law WY, Kuo CJ, et al. The diagnostic accuracy of 256-row computed tomographic angiography compared with invasive coronary angiography in patients with suspected coronary artery disease. *Eur Heart J* 2010; 31: 1916-1923.

[3] Rybicki F, Otero H, Steigner M, et al. Initial evaluation of coronary images from 320-detector row computed tomography. *Int J Cardiovasc Imaging* 2008; 24:535-546.

[4] Dewey ME, Deissenrieder ZF, Laule M, et al. Noninvasive coronary angiography by 320-row computed tomography with lower radiation exposure and maintained

diagnostic accuracy: comparison of results with cardiac catheterization in a head-to-head pilot investigation. *Circulation* 2009;120:867-875.

[5] Hausleiter J, Meyer T, Hermann F et al. Estimated radiation dose associated with cardiac CT angiography. *JAMA* 2009; 301(5):500–507.

[6] Alkadhi H, Leschka S. Radiation dose of cardiac computed tomography-what has been achieved and what needs to be done. *Eur Radiol* 2011; 21: 505-509.

[7] Deetjen A, Mollmann S, Conradi G, et al. Use of automatic exposure control in multislice computed tomography of the coronaries: comparison of 16-slice and 64-slice scanner with conventional coronary angiography. *Heart* 2007; 93: 1040-1043.

[8] Gustein A, Dev D, Cheng V, et al. Algorithm for radiation dose reduction with helical dual source coronary computed tomography angiography in clinical practice. *J Cardiovasc Comput Tomogr* 2008; 2: 311-322.

[9] Hausleiter J, Meyer T, Hadamitzky M, et al. Radiation dose estimates from cardiac multislice computed tomography in daily practice: impact of different scanning protocols on effective dose estimates. *Circulation* 2006; 113: 1305-1310.

[10] Sun Z, Ng KH. Multislice CT angiography in cardiac imaging. Part III: radiation dose and dose reduction. *Singapore Med J* 2010; 51:374-380.

[11] Tsapaki V, Rehani M. Dose measurement in CT facility. *Biomed Imaging Interve J* 2007; 3: e43.

[12] Morin L, Gerber TC, McCollough CH. Radiation dose in computed tomography of the heart. *Circulation* 2003; 107:917-922.

[13] Suzuki A, Suzuki MN. Use of a pencil-shaped ionization chamber for measurement of exposure resulting from a computed tomography scan. *Med Phys* 1978; 5:536–539.

[14] International Electrotechnical Commission. Medical Electrical Equipment. Part 2–44: Particular Requirements for the Safety of X-ray Equipment for Computed Tomography. *IEC publication* No. 60601–2-44. International Electrotechnical Commission (IEC) Central Office: Geneva, Switzerland, 2002.

[15] International Commission on Radiological Protection. *Recommendations of the ICRP,* publication 26. Pergamon, Oxford, (2007).

[16] Bongartz G, Golding SJ, Jurik AJ, et al. European guidelines for multislice computed tomography: *report EUR 16262 EN 2004.* Luxembourg: European Commission, 2004.

[17] Morin RL. Monte Carlo simulation in the radiological sciences. *Boca Raton,* FL: CRC Press; 1988.

[18] Sun Z, Ng KH. Prospective versus retrospective ECG-gated multislice CT coronary angiography: A systematic review of radiation dose and diagnostic accuracy. *Eur J Radiol* 2012; 81: e94-e100.

[19] Hendel RC, Budoff MJ, Cardella JF, et al. ACC/AHA/ACR/ASE/ASNC/HRS/NASCI /RSNA/SAIP/SCAI/SCCT/SCMR/SIR2008 key data elements and definitions for cardiac imaging. *J Am Coll Cardiol* 2009;53:91-124.

[20] Kalra MK, Maher MM, Toth TL, et al. Techniques and applications of automatic tube current modulation for CT. *Radiology* 2004; 233: 649-657.

[21] Xu L, Zhang Z. Coronary CT angiography with low radiation dose. *Int J Cardiovasc Imaging* 2010; 26:17-25.

[22] Suess, C., and X. Y. Chen. 2002. Dose optimization in pediatric CT: current technology and future innovations. *Pediatr Radiol* 32: 729-734.

[23] Herzog C, Mulvihill DM, Nguyen SA, et al. Pediatric cardiovascular CT angiography: radiation dose reduction using automatic tube current modulation. *AJR Am J Roentgenol* 2008; 190: 1232-1240.

[24] Wang J, Duan X, Christner JA, et al. Radiation dose reduction to the breast in thoracic CT: comparison of bismuth shielding, organ-based tube current modulation, and use of a globally decreased tube current. *Med Phys* 2011; 38: 6084-6092.

[25] Achenbach S, Anders K, Kalender WA. Dual-source cardiac computed tomography: image quality and dose considerations. *Eur Radiol* 2008; 18:1188–1198.

[26] Abada HT, Larchez C, Daoud B et al. MDCT of the bcoronary arteries: feasibility of low-dose CT with ECG-pulsed tube current modulation to reduce radiation dose. *AJR Am J Roentgenol* 2006; 186(6 Suppl 2):S387–S390.

[27] Jakobs TF, Becker CR, Ohnesorge B et al. Multislice helical CT of the heart with retrospective EKG gating: reduction of radiation exposure by EKG-controlled tube current modulation. *Eur Radiol* 2002; 12(5):1081–1086.

[28] Yerramasu A, Venuraju S, Atwal S, et al. Radiation dose of CT coronary angiography in clinical practice: objective evaluation of strategies for dose optimization. *Eur J Radiol* 2012; 81: 1555-1561.

[29] Yang CC, Mok GS, Law WY, et al. Potential dose reduction of optimal ECG-controlled tube current modulation for 256-slice CT coronary angiography. *Acad Radiol* 2011; 18: 731-737.

[30] Leschka S, Stolzmann P, Schmid FT et al. Low kilovoltage cardiac dual-source CT: attenuation, noise, and radiation dose. *Eur Radiol* 2008; 18:1809–1817.

[31] Park EA, Lee W, Kang JH, Yin YH, Chung JW, Park JH. The image quality and radiation dose of 100-kVp versus 120-kVp ECG-gated 16-slice CT coronary angiography. *Korean J Radiol* 2009; 10:235-243.

[32] Pflederer T, Rudofsky L, Ropers D, et al. Image quality in a low radiation exposure protocol for retrospectively ECG-gated coronary CT angiography. *AJR Am J Roentgenol* 2009; 192:1045-1050.

[33] Blankstein R, Bolen MA, Pale R, et al. Use of 100 kV versus 120 kV in cardiac dual source computed tomography: effect on radiation dose and image quality. *Int J Cardiovasc Imaging* 2011; 27: 579-586.

[34] Bischoff B, Hein FN, Meyer F, et al. Impact of reduced tube voltage on CT angiography and radiation dose: Results of the PROTECTION I Study. *J Am Coll Cardiol Imaging* 2009;2:940-6.

[35] Schoepf UJ, Becker CR, Ohnesorge BM, Yucel EK. CT of coronary artery disease. *Radiology* 2004;232:18 –37.

[36] McCollough C, Primak A, Saba O, et al. Dose performance of a 64-channel dual-source CT scanner. *Radiology* 2007;243(3):775–84.

[37] Primak AN, McCollough CH, Bruesewitz MR, et al. Relationship between noise, dose, and pitch in cardiac multi-detector row CT. *Radiographics* 2006;26(6):1785–94.

[38] Ketelsen D, Thomas C, Werner M, et al. Dual-source computed tomography: estimation of radiation exposure of ECG-gated and ECG-triggered coronary angiography. *Eur J Radiol* 2010; 73: 274-279.

[39] Brodoefel H, Burgstahler C, Tsiflokas I, et al. Dual-source CT: effect of heart rate, heart rate variability, and calcification on image quality and diagnostic accuracy. *Radiology* 2008; 247: 346-355.

[40] Johnson TR, Nikolaou K, Wintersperger BJ, et al. Dual-source CT cardiac imaging: initial experience. *Eur Radiol* 2006; 16:1409–1415.

[41] Donnino R, Jacobs JE, Doshi JV, et al. Dual-source versus single-source cardiac CT angiography: comparison of diagnostic image quality. *AJR Am J Roentgenol* 2009; 192: 1051-1056.

[42] Achenbach S, Marwan M, Ropers D, et al. Coronary computed tomography angiography with a consistent dose below 1 mSv using prospectively electrocardiogram-triggered high-pitch spiral acquisition. *Eur Heart J;* 2010;31:340-6.

[43] Lell MM, Marvan M, Schepis T, et al. Prospectively ECG-triggered high-pitch spiral acquisition for coronary CT angiography using dual source CT: technique and initial experience. *Eur Radiol* 2009; 19:2576-2583.

[44] Sommer WH, Schenzle JC, Becker CR et al. Saving dose in triple-rule-out computed tomography examination using a high-pitch dual spiral technique. *Invest Radiol* 2009; 45:64–71.

[45] Lell M, Hinkmann F, Anders K et al. High-pitch electrocardiogram-triggered computed tomography of the chest: initial results. *Invest Radiol* 2009; 44:728–733.

[46] Leschka S, Stolzmann P, Desbiolles L et al. Diagnostic accuracy of high-pitch dual-source CT for the assessment of coronary stenoses: first experience. *Eur Radiol* 2009;19:2896–2903.

[47] Alkadhi H, Stolzmann P, Desbiolles L et al. Low-dose, 128-slice, dual-source CT coronary angiography: accuracy and radiation dose of the high-pitch and the step-and-shoot mode. *Heart* 2010; 96:933–938.

[48] Husmann L, Valenta I, Gaemperli O et al. Feasibility of low-dose coronary CT angiography: first experience with prospective ECG-gating. *Eur Heart J* 2008; 29(2):191–197.

[49] Shuman WP, Branch KR, May JM et al. Prospective versus retrospective ECG gating for 64-detector CT of the coronary arteries: comparison of image quality and patient radiation dose. *Radiology* 2008; 248(2):431–437.

[50] Hirai N, Horiguchi J, Fujioka C et al. Prospective versus retrospective ECG-gated 64-detector coronary CT angiography: assessment of image quality, stenosis, and radiation dose. *Radiology* 2008; 248(2):424–430.

[51] Earls JP, Berman EL, Urban BA et al. Prospectively gated transverse coronary CT angiography versus retrospectively gated helical technique: improved image quality and reduced radiation dose. *Radiology* 2008; 246(3):742–753.

[52] Lu B, Lu J, Sun M, et al. Comparison of diagnostic accuracy and radiation dose between prospective triggering and retrospective gated coronary angiography by dual-source computed tomography. *Am J Cardiol* 2011; 107: 1278-1284.

[53] Huang B, Li J, Law MWM, Zhang J, Shen Y, Khong PL. Radiation dose and cancer risk in retrospectively and prospectively ECG-gated coronary angiography using 64-slice multidetector CT. *Br J Radiol* 2010; 83: 152-158.

[54] Stolzmann P, Goetti R, Baumueller S, et al. Prospective and retrospective ECG-gating for CT coronary angiography perform similarly accurate at low heart rates. *Eur J Radiol* 2011; 79: 85-91.

[55] von Ballmoos WM, Haring B, Juillert P, Alkadhi H. Meta-analysis: diagnostic performance of low-radiation-dose coronary computed tomography angiography. *Ann Intern Med* 2011; 154: 413-420.

[56] Sun Z, Ng KH. Diagnostic value of coronary CT angiography with prospective ECG-gating in the diagnosis of coronary artery disease: A systematic review and meta-analysis. *Int J Cardiovasc Imaging*2012; 28: 2109-2119..

[57] Pelliccia F, Pasceri V, Evangelista A, et al. Diagnostic accuracy of 320-row computed tomography as compared with invasive coronary angiography in unselected, consecutive patients with suspected coronary artery disease. *Int J Cardiovasc Imaging* DOI 10.1007/s10554-012-0095-4

[58] Nasis A, Leung MC, Antonis P, et al. Diagnostic accuracy of noninvasive coronary angiography with 320-detector row computed tomography. *Am J Cardiol* 2010; 106: 1429-1435.

[59] Lee TY, Chhem RK. Impact of new technologies on dose reduction in CT. *Eur J Radiol* 2010; 76: 28-35.

[60] Leipsic J, Heilbron BG, Hague C. Iterative reconstruction for coronary CT angiography: findings its way. *Int J Cardiovasc Imaging* 2012; 28: 613-620.

[61] Gosling O, Loader R, Venables P, et al. A comparison of radiation doses between state-of-the-art multislice CT coronary angiography with iterative reconstruction, multislice CT coronary angiography with standard filtered back-projection and invasive diagnostic coronary angiography. *Heart* 2010; 96: 922-926.

Chapter 4

64-Slice Coronary CT Angiography in Coronary Artery Disease: A Systematic Review of Diagnostic Value, Image Quality and Radiation Dose

Abstract

To perform a systematic review of the diagnostic value, image quality and radiation dose of 64-slice coronary CT angiography in the diagnosis of coronary artery disease when compared to invasive coronary angiography. A search of PUBMED and MEDLINE databases was conducted to identify studies investigating the diagnostic value of 64-slice coronary CT angiography in the diagnosis of coronary artery disease. Diagnostic value of coronary CT angiography was compared to invasive coronary angiography and analyzed at patient-, vessel- and segment-based analysis. Factors affecting diagnostic value and image quality were identified. Twenty-two studies met selection criteria and were included for analysis. Pooled estimates and 95% confidence interval (CI) of sensitivity, specificity, positive predictive value and negative predictive value of 64-slice coronary CT angiography were 98% (95% CI: 96%, 99%), 89% (95% CI: 86%, 91%), 92% (95% CI: 90%, 94%), and 97% (95% CI: 95%, 98%), according to the patient-based assessment. The mean values of sensitivity, specificity, positive predictive value and negative predictive value of 64-slice coronary CT angiography were 92% (95% CI: 88%, 96%), 92% (95% CI: 87%, 99%), 78% (95% CI: 62%, 93%) and 98% (95% CI: 97%, 99%) according to the vessel-based assessment; 88% (95% CI: 84%, 93%), 96% (95% CI: 95%, 97%), 74%(95% CI: 65%, 82%) and 99% (95% CI: 98%, 99%) according to the segment-based assessment, respectively. Radiation dose of 64-slice CT coronary angiography was reported in 50% of the studies, with mean value of 13.5 mSv for males, which is significantly lower than the 18.5 mSv for females. The main factor that affected image quality was severe calcification, which decreased the diagnostic accuracy and image quality at segment-based analysis. Sixty-four-slice coronary CT angiography has a high diagnostic value in the diagnosis of coronary artery disease. Severe coronary calcification seems to be the major factor affecting the diagnostic performance of coronary CT angiography.

Keywords: 64-slice CT, coronary artery disease, coronary CT angiography, diagnostic value, image quality, radiation dose

4.1. Introduction

Coronary artery disease (CAD) is the leading cause of death in developed countries [1]. The standard of reference for diagnosis of CAD is still invasive coronary angiography, with the advantage of superior spatial resolution and temporal resolution. However, its diagnostic value has been challenged due to its invasiveness and procedure-related complications by the introduction of coronary CT angiography performed with multislice CT scanners. Previous reports showed that coronary CT angiography is a promising technique with the increase of detector rows from 4-slice to 16-slice and 64-slice scanners [2-10]. With the increase of number of detectors, more coronary segments were evaluable, and the sensitivity for a significant coronary stenosis in evaluable segment was reported to increase [8-10]. However, diagnostic value of coronary CT angiography with early generations of multislice CT scanners such as 4-slice and 16-slice was still limited and has not reached the accuracy as that of invasive coronary angiography. Preliminary data showed that 64-slice coronary CT angiography is more sensitive and specific than earlier 4-slice and 16-slice CT in the diagnosis of CAD [10-12]. Currently there is a lack of data for a systematic analysis of the diagnostic value of 64-slice coronary CT angiography in coronary artery disease. Therefore, the aim of this chapter was to perform a systematic review of 64-slice coronary CT angiography in the detection of CAD with regard to the diagnostic value in comparison to invasive coronary angiography, based on the available studies in the literature.

4.2. Materials and Methods

4.2.1. Criteria for Data Selection and Literature Screening

A search of PUBMED and MEDLINE databases for English literature was performed for studies describing the diagnostic value of 64-slice coronary CT angiography in CAD compared to invasive coronary angiography. The articles must be peer-reviewed and published in English language. The keywords used in searching for relevant articles were: 64-slice CT and coronary artery stenosis/disease; 64-slice coronary CT angiography; 64-slice coronary CT angiography in CAD; 64-slice CT in CAD.

The search was limited to reports on human subjects and excluded case reports, conference abstracts, review articles, in vitro studies and articles investigating the coronary stent or bypass graft treatments. Exclusion criteria were also extended to the investigations performed with 64-more slice CT techniques or methods, electron beam CT. The search of literature was selected to range from 2004 to 2012 (June 2012), as 64-slice CT was first introduced into clinical practice in 2004 [13]. In addition, the reference lists of identified articles were checked to obtain additional relevant articles.

Prospective and retrospective studies were included if they met all of the following criteria: (a) patients undergoing 64-slice CT angiography with use of retrospective ECG-gating, as studies performed with prospective ECG-triggering were discussed in Chapter 10; (b) studies included at least 10 patients; (c) assessment or comparison of 64-slice CT angiography with coronary angiography was focused on the visualization of coronary arteries and detection or exclusion of coronary artery stenosis; (d) diagnostic value of 64-slice CT angiography was addressed when compared to invasive coronary angiography in terms of sensitivity, specificity, positive predictive value (PPV), negative predictive value (NPV), either according to patients-based, vessel-based or segments-based assessment.

4.2.2. Data Extraction

Data were extracted repeatedly based on study design and procedure techniques. The reviewer looked for the following characteristics in each study: year of publication; number of participants in the study; mean age; mean heart rate; number of male patients; mean body mass index (BMI); number of patients receiving β–blockers; prevalence of suspected or known CAD; assessable coronary segments in each study; image quality assessment (qualitative or quantitative analysis); coronary artery calcium scores; radiation dose associated with 64-slice coronary CT angiography; diagnostic accuracy of 64-slice CT when compared to invasive coronary angiography in terms of the sensitivity, specificity, PPV, NPV and main factors affecting the visualization of coronary arteries or diagnostic performance. All diagnostic accuracy estimates referred to segment/vessel/patient-based assessment. Sensitivity, specificity, PPV and NPV were calculated with use of the following equations:

$$\text{Sensitivity} = \frac{\text{Number of TP}}{\text{Number of TP} + \text{Number of FN}}$$

$$\text{Specificity} = \frac{\text{Number of TN}}{\text{Number of TN} + \text{Number of FP}}$$

$$\text{PPV} = \frac{\text{Number of TP}}{\text{Number of TP} + \text{Number of FP}}$$

$$\text{NPV} = \frac{\text{Number of TN}}{\text{Number of TN} + \text{Number of FN}}$$

TP-true positive, TN-true negative, FP-false positive, FN-false negative.

4.2.3. Definition of Coronary Segments and Stenosis

Significant stenosis was defined as more than 50% stenosis of the coronary artery lumen which is hemodynamically significant. High-grade stenosis was defined as more than 75% stenosis. In this chapter, the diagnostic value of 64-slice coronary CT angiography in CAD was analysed based on more than 50% stenosis. Coronary artery segments were numbered as defined by the American Heart Association [14]. Assessment of coronary artery was based on variable descriptions as some investigators listed the segments, while others described the portion of the arteries evaluated in terms of numbered segments. The 15/17-segment assessment is commonly used by investigators in these studies comparing 64-slice coronary CT angiography with invasive coronary angiography.

4.2.4. Statistical Analysis

All of the data were entered into SPSS (version 19.0) for analysis. Sensitivity, specificity, PPV and NPV estimates for each study were combined across studies using one sample test. Between-study heterogeneity of the sensitivity, specificity, PPV and NPV estimates was tested using the Mantel-Haenszel Chi-squared test with n-1 degree of freedom (n is the number of studies). Comparison was performed by Chi Square test to test if there is any significant difference regarding the diagnostic value of coronary CT angiography in CAD, between segment-based assessment, vessel-based assessment or patient-based assessment. Statistical hypotheses (2-tailed) were tested at the 5% level of significance.

4.3. Results

4.3.1. General Information

Twenty-two studies met criteria for inclusion in the analysis [15-36]. Studies reported from the same institutions or research groups were still included in the analysis, as long as the recruited data consisted of different risk groups or clinical assessment of coronary CT angiography was investigated with a focus on different aspects. There were 9 studies involving multiple comparisons in different groups, with 5 studies (22 comparisons) at patient-based assessment; 2 studies (7 comparisons) at vessel-based assessment and 8 studies (34 comparisons) at segment-based assessment dealing with the diagnostic value of 64-slice coronary CT angiography in CAD based on effect of different coronary calcium scores [15, 16, 19, 26, 28, 31, 32], body mass index [19], and variable heart rates [29, 30]. Figure 4.1 is the flow chart showing the search strategy to obtain these eligible references.

Table 4.1 shows the study characteristics in each article reviewed. The number of patients enrolled in these studies ranged from 35 to 208. There were 6 studies involving more than 100 cases [25, 26, 30-32, 36]. Of 22 studies retrieved, all were performed on single-source 64-slice scanners with spatial resolution of 165 ms to 200 ms, while studies performed on dual-source CT scanner were excluded as a detailed analysis of the diagnostic value of dual-source CT was presented in Chapter 5. Most of the coronary CT scans were performed with

Siemens scanners, while in two studies coronary CT angiography was done on Toshiba scanner and one study was performed on GE Healthcare.

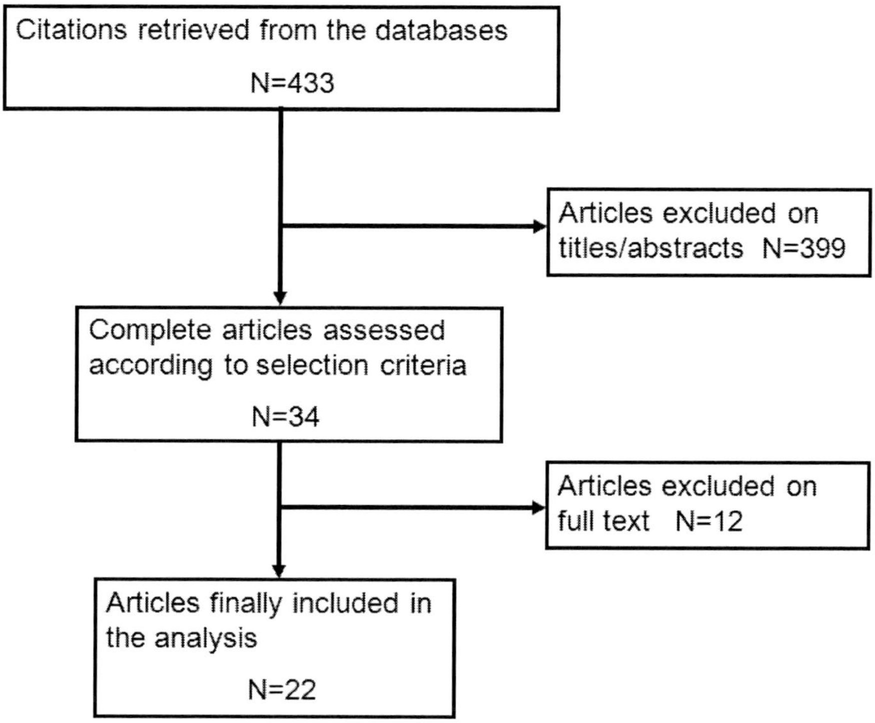

Figure 4.1. Flow chart showing the searching strategy to obtain eligible references on 64-slice coronary CT angiography.

Of all studies reviewed, it was found that the male patients were most commonly affected with CAD, with pooled estimate and 95% confidence interval (CI) being 65% (95% CI: 58%, 73%). β-blocker was used in 13 studies (59%) and the mean value and 95% CI was 55% (95% CI: 36%, 74%). The mean heart rate of patients during scan ranged from 58 to 90 beats per minute (bpm) across studies (median, 61 bpm). The percentage of assessable segments was available in 17 studies with the mean value and 95% CI being 96% (95% CI: 94%, 97%). Coronary artery calcium scores were reported in 7 studies with the mean value and 95% CI of 322 (95% CI: 235, 410).

Of four studies, 64-slice coronary CT angiography in CAD was investigated for different degree of coronary stenosis (>50% vs 75%) [16], different BMI ranges [19], and variable heart rates [29, 30]. However, comparison could not be performed due to limited data and different method of analysis (patient-based or segment-based), although the sensitivity of 64-slice coronary CT angiography in the evaluation of >75% stenosis showed slightly higher than that in >50% stenosis (80% vs 73%); and application of heart rate control significantly improved the diagnostic performance of 64-slice coronary CT angiography. In patients with large BMI (>30 kg/m^2), diagnostic accuracy was reduced when compared to the overall accuracy of 64-slice coronary CT angiography in patients with a normal BMI.

Table 4.1 Study characteristics of 64-slice coronary CT angiography in coronary artery disease

Studies	Year of publication	Detector collimation	No. Patients	No. of cases β blocker %	Mean age (yrs)	No. of Male	HR	BMI	Assessable segments (%)	Calcium score	Effective dose (mSv)
Mollet et al (15)	2005	2x32x0.6	52	73	59.6± 12.1	34	57.8 ±6.8	NA	97	231 (15-736)	15.2:21.4 (M:F)
Leber et al (16)	2005	64x0.6	59	35	64± 10	NS	62 ± 13	NA	100	Severely/non, moderate	10-14
Leschka et al (17)	2005	64x0.6	67	60	60.1±10.5	50	66.3± 14.7	NA	100	NA	NA
Plass et al (18)	2005	2x32x0.6	50	NA	66±8	39	65±11	NA	97	NA	NA
Raff et al (19)	2005	2x32x0.6	70	NA	59±11	53	65±10	30±5	88	326 ± 472	13:18 (M:F)
Ehara et al (20)	2006	64x0.6	69	22	67±11	52	71.8± 13.2	NA	92	NA	NA
Nikolaou et al (21)	2006	2x32x0.6	72	NA	64±10	59	61±9	NA	90	NA	NA
Pugliese et al (22)	2006	2x32x0.6	35	NA	61±10	21	58±6	NA	97	NA	15:20 (M:F)
Schuijf et al (23)	2006	64x0.5	60	72	60±11	14	60±11	NA	99	423±868	NA
Ropers et al (24)	2006	64x0.6	84	74	58±10	52	59±9	29±5	96	NA	7.45:10.24 (M:F)
Shabestari et al (25)	2007	64x0.6	143	89	63±10	103	65	NA	96	0-1213	NA
Meijboom et al (26) *	2007	64x0.6	104	86	58±7/ 59±10	23/52	60±8	25.8±3.6 /26.5±3.7	NS	473.9±738.2/44 0±513.6	15.2:21.4 (M:F)
Muhlenbruch et al (27)	2007	64x0.6	51	NA	58.5±7.9	39	61±7.7	NA	95	NA	13.6:17.3 (M:F)
Oncel et al (28)	2007	2x32x0.6	80	53	56	61	58±10	NA	100	NA	NA
Achenbach et al (29) ##	2008	64x0.6	45/55	0/90	65±11/ 65±11	17/23	70±15/ 60±8	NA	82/93	NA	13±2.7/12±2.0

Studies	Year of publication	Detector collimation	No. Patients	No. of cases β blocker %	Mean age (yrs)	No. of Male	HR	BMI	Assessable segments (%)	Calcium score	Effective dose (mSv)
Brodoefel et al (30)	2008	64x0.6	102	62	62±10	82	68.2± 13.1	27.5±4.1	98	226.5	NA
Diederichsen et al (31)	2009	64x0.625	109	NA	63±11	58	NA	27±4	NA	267	21.3
Palumbo et al (32) #	2009	2x32x0.6	200	NA	57±13	169	56.8±8.8	26.8±3.5	NA	313±606	NA
Yang et al (33)	2009	64x0.5	60	0	58.7±12.9	37	90±13.1	24.5±3.6	97	NA	14.5±4.3
Wehrschuetz et al (34)	2010	64x0.6	37	0	64.3±2.3	22	73.4±1.7	NA	92	NA	NA
Romagnoli et al (35)	2010	64x0.6	64	NA	65±10	38	63	NA	NA	NA	NA
Cademartiri et al (36)	2010	64x0.6	208	NA	48±11	57	59.4±6.7	29±5	NA	NA	15:21 (M:F)

*two groups (low risk and high risk patients) were included; # five groups based on calcium scores; ## no heart rate control and heart rate control groups, M-male, F-female, NA-not available.

4.3.2. Image Quality Assessment

Subjective assessment of coronary CT angiography images was conducted in 15 studies by two observers who were blinded to the results of invasive coronary angiography, with use of 3- or 4-point scoring scale applied in 10 studies. Only one observer was involved in the evaluation of image quality in 5 studies, while in the remaining two studies, details of observer assessment were not available. In contrast, in more than half of the studies (59%), invasive coronary angiographic images were evaluated by one observer, while in the remaining 9 studies, two observers were involved in the assessment of angiographic images.

Quantitative assessment of image quality was only conducted in one study with use of contrast-to-noise ratio to determine the image quality [16].

4.3.3. Radiation Dose

Radiation dose was reported in 11 studies, while in the remaining studies, information on radiation exposure associated with coronary CT angiography was not available. The mean radiation dose for males was 13.5 ±2.7 mSv, which is significantly lower than that measured for females, which is 18.5 ±3.9 mSv. A tube voltage of 120 kVp was consistently used throughout these studies, regardless of the BMI ranges, and no dose-saving strategies were applied in these 64-slice coronary CT angiography examinations.

4.3.4. Coronary Segments Included in the Analysis

Although the AHA classification system was used in all of the 22 studies, different coronary segments were included for analysis among these studies. A 17-segment AHA system was used in 8 studies, followed by 15-segment method in 6 studies, and 13- and 11-segment method in one study each. Details of the coronary segments were not available in the remaining 6 studies.

4.3.5. Prevalence of Suspected or Know CAD

Prevalence of CAD in these studies was variable according to this review; we categorized it into suspected and known CAD. Patients suspected of CAD indicate that the patients presented with clinical symptoms such as typical or atypical chest pain, elevated ST, and they were recommended for coronary angiography for confirmation of presence of the lesion (stenosis/occlusion). The mean value and 95% CI of suspected CAD was 63% (95% CI: 44%, 82%). In contrast, known CAD refers to these patients which were confirmed to suffer from coronary artery disease (presence of stenosis or occlusion) by invasive coronary angiography. This analysis showed that high-risk or known CAD ranged from 17% to 88%, with the mean value and 95% CI being 53% (95% CI: 40%, 67%). No significant difference was found when compared the prevalence of low risk CAD or suspected CAD with that of high risk or known CAD ($p>0.05$).

4.3.6. Diagnostic Value of 64-Slice Coronary CT Angiography: Patient-Based Analysis

Of 22 studies, evaluation of 64-slice coronary CT angiography in CAD on patient-based assessment was available in 15 studies. No statistical heterogeneity was found for these analyses according to patient-based assessment among these studies, so the pooled estimates across studies were used to demonstrate the diagnostic performance. Pooled estimates and 95% CI of the sensitivity, specificity, PPV and NPV of 64-slice coronary CT angiography were 98% (95% CI: 96%, 99%), 89% (95% CI: 86%, 91%), 92% (95% CI: 90%, 94%), and 97% (95% CI: 95%, 98%) (Figs 4.2, 4.3).

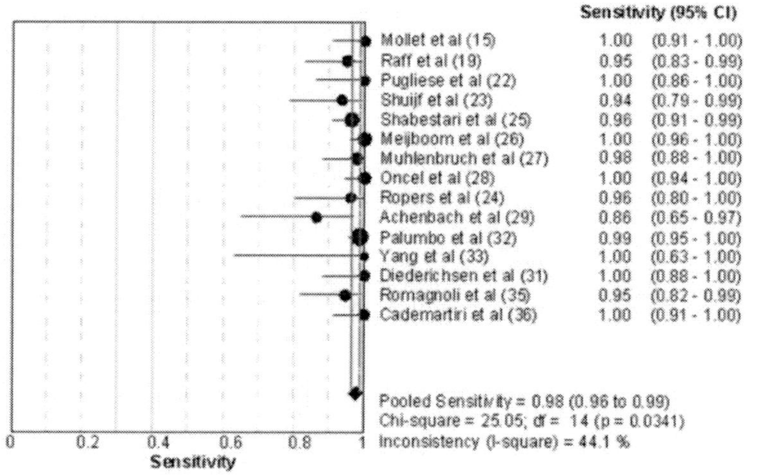

Figure 4.2. Plot of pooled sensitivity of 64-slice coronary CT angiography compared to invasive coronary angiography in 15 studies based on patient-based assessment. CI-confidence interval.

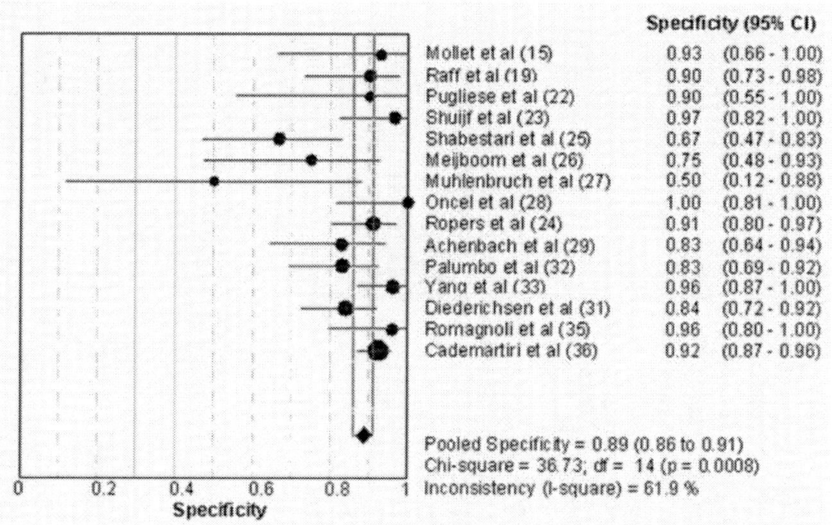

Figure 4.3. Plot of pooled specificity of 64-slice coronary CT angiography compared to invasive coronary angiography in 15 studies based on patient-based assessment. CI-confidence interval.

4.3.7. Diagnostic Value of 64-Slice Coronary CT Angiography: Vessel-and Segment-Based Analysis

Severe heterogeneity/inconsistency was noticed at the vessel-based and segment-based assessment levels ($p<0.05$), so pooling was avoided, and only the mean values across these studies were described. The mean values of sensitivity, specificity, PPV and NPV were 92% (95% CI: 88%, 96%), 92% (95% CI: 87%, 99%), 78% (95% CI: 62%, 93%) and 98% (95% CI: 97%, 99%), according to vessel-based assessment which was available in 8 studies; 88% (95% CI: 84%, 93%), 96% (95% CI: 95%, 97%), 74% (95% CI: 65%, 82%) and 99% (95% CI: 98%, 99%), according to segment-based assessment, which was reported in 15 studies.

4.3.8. Effect of Coronary Calcium Scores on Diagnostic Value

Diagnostic accuracy of 64-slice coronary CT angiography in CAD was influenced by the presence of calcification and its relationship to the degree of coronary calcium scores was investigated in three studies with 12 comparisons according to patient-based assessment; in seven studies with 24 comparisons according to segment-based analysis. Table 4.2 shows the mean values and 95% CI of 64-slice coronary CT angiography in studies comparing the different coronary calcium scores and corresponding diagnostic value. There was no significant difference between low, moderate and high coronary calcium scores in terms of diagnostic performance at the level of patient-based evaluation, however, significant differences were found in the specificity, PPV and NPV according to segment-based analysis ($p<0.05$), indicating the significant effect of severe calcification on the diagnostic value of 64-slice coronary CT angiography.

Table 4.2. Mean value of sensitivity, specificity, PPV and NPV of 64-slice coronary CT angiography according to different coronary calcium scores

Assessment levels		Sensitivity (95% CI)	Specificity (95% CI)	Positive predictive value (95% CI)	Negative predictive value (95% CI)
Patient-based assessment	Low CAC	95% (90%, 100%)	87% (59%, 100%)	87% (59%, 100%)	97% (88%, 100%)
	Moderate CAC	100%	87% (61%, 100%)	100%	83.5%
	High CAC	98% (88%, 100%)	89% (57%, 100%)	98% (88%, 100%)	100%
Segment-based assessment	Low CAC	91% (84%, 98%)	98% (96%, 99%)	81% (68%, 94%)	99% (99%, 100%)
	Moderate CAC	91% (81%, 99%)	92% (87%, 98%)	73% (60%, 86%)	98% (97%, 99%)
	High CAC	92% (85%, 99%)	85% (74%, 95%)	70% (53%, 88%)	98% (96%, 99%)

CAC-coronary calcium score.

Discussion

This chapter shows that 64-slice coronary CT angiography has high diagnostic accuracy in the diagnosis of CAD, according to patient-based, vessel-based or segment-based analysis.

In particular, a very high negative predictive value (>97%) has been achieved with 64-slice coronary CT angiography indicating that this technique can be used as a reliable screening tool for patients with suspected CAD.

In comparison to earlier scanners such as 4-slice and 16-slice CT, 64-slice coronary CT angiography has demonstrated significant improvements in the assessment of coronary artery branches. Studies performed on the 16-slice CT scanners in the detection of CAD showed that the sensitivity of coronary CT angiography decreased when assessing the distal coronary segments due to limited spatial and temporal resolution [12]. In comparison to 16-slice CT scanners, the current 64-slice scanner has increased slices per gantry rotation and fast gantry speed (330 ms vs 375ms), which translate into superior spatial resolution (0.5 mm vs 0.75 mm) and temporal resolution (165ms vs 188 ms). The reduction in voxel size allows acquisition of isotropic volume data and makes distinction between hypointense soft plaque and contrast-enhanced blood more evident. Moreover, more coronary segments can be assessed with 64-slice CT angiography with the percentage of assessable segments being higher than that from 16-slice scanners. Percentage of assessable segments in this analysis was 96%, which is significantly higher than that of 16-and 4-slice scanners, which is 92% and 74%, according to a previous meta-analysis [37].

Recent studies have reported that two major limitations for affecting the coronary CT angiography evaluation of coronary artery segments are motion artefacts and severe coronary calcifications. In order to reduce motion artefacts, β-blockers were commonly used prior to CT examination, even if in the 64-slice scanners, as shown in this analysis. Consistent use of beta-blocking agents before the scan to keep patients' heart rates below 60 bpm could produce better results in some studies. This is observed in this analysis, as the mean heart rate is less than 65 bpm during coronary CT angiography in 68% of the studies, and this indicates the necessity of controlling heart rate to ensure acquisition of diagnostic image quality. The latest development of dual-source CT has been reported to improve temporal resolution when compared to early 64-slice scanners, and coronary arteries were visualized without motion artefacts at any heart rate and beta blocker utilization could be discarded [38, 39]. Initial experience on dual-source CT showed the advantages of imaging patients with high heart rates and reduction of occurrence of motion artefacts in comparison to earlier 64-slice scanners [38], although further studies need to be performed to establish the diagnostic accuracy of dual-source CT in the diagnosis of CAD. Dual-source CT coronary angiography has been increasingly used in clinical practice, and the analysis of its diagnostic value and image quality will be discussed in chapter 5.

Another common factor that affects evaluation of coronary artery lumen is the presence of extensive calcification. Similar to 4-slice and 16-slice CT, extensive artery calcifications are a frequent source of impairing vessel assessment, even with 64-slice CT, although the degree of artefacts due to partial volume effects seem to be less severe. Severe calcification obscures coronary lumen and can lead to overestimation of the severity of the lesions due to blooming artefacts, making quantification of the degree of coronary artery stenosis difficult. The interference of calcification with assessment of coronary artery lumen was reported in seven studies, and the analysis showed that the specificity, PPV and NPV was significantly decreased with the increase of the calcium score, indicating the relatively high false positive cases resulting from extensive calcification. Thus, caution should be considered in imaging patients with severe calcifications.

BMI seems to be another factor that may affect the diagnostic accuracy of 64-slice coronary CT angiography. This was investigated in one study which demonstrated the relationship between BMI and diagnostic value of 64-slice coronary CT angiography [19]. Relevant research has been performed to investigate the relationship between body weight/BMI and image noise for reduction of radiation exposure without loss of diagnostic information in CT scanning protocols [40, 41]. Yoshimura et al recently reported that image noise correlated well with body weight in coronary CT angiography [40]. Therefore, relationship between radiation dose, image noise and diagnostic accuracy need to be further investigated to minimize radiation dose while maintaining adequate diagnostic information for clinical investigation of coronary artery disease.

There are some limitations in this analysis that should be addressed. Firstly, publication bias may have affected the results as non-English references were excluded. Secondly, lack of uniform criteria of assessment is another limitation inherent in most of the studies analysed. Inclusion of variable numbers of coronary segments makes the analysis and comparison of coronary CT angiography performance difficult. Not all of the studies provided detailed information about the diagnostic value of 64-slice coronary CT angiography. Assessment of four main coronary branches was only reported in a small number of studies, thus, a systematic analysis was not conducted. Finally, radiation dose was only reported in half of the studies. In addition, other dose parameters such as volume CT dose index or dose length product were not available in all of the studies. The increase in dose estimates with 64-slice CT when compared to 4-and 16-slice scanners is due to the higher spatial and temporal resolution achieved with the current CT scanner technology and therefore, thus radiation dose of 64-slice CT in cardiac imaging deserves to be investigated.

In conclusion, this chapter demonstrates that 64-slice coronary CT angiography has a high diagnostic value in the diagnosis of coronary artery disease, with very high assessable segments and negative predictive value achieved. For patients with extensive calcifications in the coronary lumen or coronary artery stenoses, diagnostic performance of 64-slice coronary CT angiography is apparently affected in the segment-based assessment. Sixty-four-slice coronary CT angiography is associated with high radiation dose, and this needs to be addressed in further studies with implementation of effective dose-saving strategies.

Acknowledgment

The author would like to thank Mr Gil Stevenson for his assistance in the statistical analysis of results.

References

[1] American Heart Association, American Stroke Association. *2002 Heart and stroke statistical update*. Dallas, TX: The American Heart Association, 2002.

[2] Nieman K, Oudkerk M, Rensing BJ, et al. Coronary angiography with multi-slice computed tomography. *Lancet* 2001; 357: 599-603.

[3] Kopp AF, Schroeder S, Kuettner A, et al. Non-invasive coronary angiography with high resolution multidetector-row computed tomography: Results in 102 patients. *Eur Heart J* 2002; 23: 1714-1725.

[4] Achenbach S, Giesler T, Ropers D, et al. Detection of coronary artery stenoses by contrast-enhanced, retrospectively electrocardiographically-gated, multislice computed tomography. *Circulation* 2001; 103: 2535-2538.

[5] Kuettner A, Trabold T, Schroeder S, et al. Noninvasive detection of coronary artery lesions using 16-detector row multislice spiral computed tomography technology: initial clinical results. *J Am Coll Cardiol* 2004; 44: 1230-1237.

[6] Nieman K, Cademartiri F, Lemos PA, et al. Reliable non-invasive coronary angiography with fast submillimeter multislice spiral computed tomography. *Circulation*; 2002; 106: 2051-2054.

[7] Mollet NR, Cademartiri F, Nieman K, et al. Multislice spiral computed tomography coronary angiography in patients with stable angina pectoris. *J Am Coll Cardiol* 2004; 43: 2265-2270.

[8] Kuettner A, Kopp AF, Schroeder S, et al. Diagnostic accuracy of multidetector computed tomography coronary angiography in patients with angiographically proved coronary artery disease. *J Am Coll Cardiol* 2004; 43: 831-839.

[9] Achenbach S, Ropers S, Pohle FK, et al. Detection of coronary artery stenoses using multi-detector CT with 16x0.75 collimation and 375ms rotation. *Eur Heart J* 2005; 26: 1978-1986.

[10] Stein PD, Beemath A, Kayali F, et al. Multidetector computed tomography for the diagnosis of coronary artery disease: a systematic review. *Am Heart J* 2006; 119: 203-216.

[11] Fine JJ, Hopkins CB, Ruff N, Newton FC. Comparison of accuracy of 64-slice cardiovascular computed tomography with coronary angiography in patients with suspected coronary artery disease. *Am J Cardiol* 2006; 97: 173-174.

[12] Kopp AF, Heuschmid M, Reimann A, et al. Advances in imaging protocols for cardiac MDCT: from 16- to 64-row multidetector computed tomography. *Eur Radiol* 2005; 15 (Suppl 5): E71-E77.

[13] Nikolaou K, Flohr T, Knez A, et al. Advances in cardiac CT imaging: 64-slice scanner. *Int J Cardiovasc Imaging* 2004; 20: 535-540.

[14] Austen WG, Edwards JE, Frye RL, et al. A reporting system on patients evaluated for coronary artery disease. Report of the Ad Hoc Committee for Grading of Coronary Artery Disease, Council on Cardiovascular Surgery, American Heart Association. *Circulation* 1975; 51: 5-40.

[15] Mollet NR, Cademartiri F, van Mieghem C, et al. High-resolution spiral computed tomography coronary angiography in patients referred for diagnostic conventional coronary angiography. *Circulation* 2005; 112: 2318-2323.

[16] Leber AW, Knez A, von Ziegler F, et al. Quantification of obstructive and non obstructive coronary lesions by 64-slice computed tomography: A comparative study with quantitative coronary angiography and intravascular ultrasound. *J Am Coll Cardiol* 2005; 46: 147-54.

[17] Leschka S, Alkadhi H, Plass A, et al. Accuracy of MSCT coronary angiography with 64-slice technology: first experience. *Eur Heart J* 2005, 26: 1482-1487.

[18] Plass A, Grunenfelder J, Leschka S, et al. Coronary artery imaging with 64-slice computed tomography from cardiac surgical perspective. *Eur J Radiol* 2006; 30: 109-116.

[19] Raff GL, Gallagher MJ, O'Neill WW, et al. Diagnostic accuracy of non-invasive coronary angiography using 64-slice spiral computed tomography. *J Am Coll Cardiol* 2005, 46: 552-557.

[20] Ehara M, Surmely JF, Kawai M, et al. Diagnostic accuracy of 64-slice computed tomography for detecting angiographically significant coronary artery stenosis in an unselected consecutive patient population: comparison with conventional invasive angiography. *Cir J* 2006; 70: 564-571.

[21] Nikolaou K, Knez A, Rist C, et al. Accuracy of 64-MDCT in the diagnosis of ischemic heart disease. *AJR Am J Roentgenol* 2006; 187: 111-117.

[22] Pugliese F, Mollet NR, Runza G, et al. Diagnostic accuracy of non-invasive 64-slice CT coronary angiography in patients with stable angina pectoris. *EurRadiol* 2006; 16: 575-582.

[23] Schuijf JD, Pundziute G, Jukema JW, et al. Diagnostic accuracy of 64-slice multislice computed tomography in the non-invasive evaluation of significant coronary artery disease. *Am J Cardiol* 2006; 98: 145-148.

[24] Ropers D, Rixe J, Anders K, et al. Usefulness of multidetector row spiral computed tomography with 64- x 0.6 mm collimation and 330-ms rotation for the noninvasive detection of significant coronary artery stenosis. *Am J Cardiol* 2006; 97: 343-348.

[25] Shabestari AA, Abdi S, Akhlaghpoor S, et al. Diagnostic performance of 64-channel multislice computed tomography in assessment of significant coronary artery disease in symptomatic subjects. *Am J Cardiol* 2007; 99: 1656-1661.

[26] Meijboom WB, Mollet NR, van Mieghem CA et al. 64-slice computed tomography coronary angiography in patients with non-ST elevation acute coronary syndrome. *Heart* 2007; 93: 1386-1392.

[27] Muhlenbruch G, Seyfarth T, Soo CS, Pregalathan N, Mahnken AH. Diagnostic value of 64-slice multi-detector row cardiac CTA in symptomatic patients. *Eur Radiol* 2007; 17: 603-609.

[28] Oncel D, Oncel G, Tastan A, Tamci B. Detection of significant coronary artery stenosis with 64-section MDCT angiography. *Eur J Radiol* 2007; 62: 394-405.

[29] Achenbach S, Ropers U, Kuettner A, et al. Randomized comparison of 64-slice single- and dual-source computed tomography coronary angiography for the detection of coronary artery disease. *JACC Cardiovasc Imaging* 2008; 1: 177-186.

[30] Brodoefel H, Reimann A, Burgstahler C, et al. Noninvasive coronary angiography using 64-slice spiral computed tomography in an unselected patient collective: effect of heart rate, heart rate variability and coronary calcifications on image quality and diagnostic accuracy. *Eur J Radiol* 2008; 66: 134-141.

[31] Diederichsen AC, Petersen H, Jensen LO, et al. Diagnostic value of cardiac 64-slice computed tomography: importance of coronary calcium. *Scan Cardiovasc J* 2009; 43: 337-344.

[32] Palumbo AA, Maffei E, Martini G, et cl. Coronary calcium score as gatekeeper for 64-slice computed tomography coronary angiography in patients with chest pain: per-segment and per-patient analysis. *Eur Radiol* 2009; 19: 2127-2135.

[33] Yang L, Zhang Z, Fan Z, et al. 64-MDCT coronary angiography of patients with atrial fibrillation: influence of heart rate on image quality and efficacy in evaluation of coronary artery disease. *AJR Am J Roentgenol* 2009; 193: 795-801.

[34] Wehrschuetz M, Wehrschuetz E, Schuchlenz H, Schaffler G. Accuracy of MSCT coronary angiography with 64 row CT scanner-facing the facts. *Clin Med Insights Cardiol* 2010; 8: 15-22.

[35] Romagnoli A, Martuscelli E, Sperandio M, et al. Role of 64-sliec cardiac computed tomography in the evaluation of patients with non-ST-elevation acute coronary syndrome. *Radio Med* 2010; 115: 341-353.

[36] Cademartiri F, Maffei E, Palumbo A, et al. Diagnostic accuracy of computed tomography coronary angiography in patients with a zero calcium score. *Eur Radiol* 2010; 20: 81-87.

[37] Sun Z, Jiang W. Diagnostic value of multislice CT angiography in coronary artery disease: A meta-analysis. *Eur J R* 2006; 60: 279-286.

[38] Flohr TG, McCollough CH, Bruder H, et al. First performance evaluation of a dual-source CT (DSCT) system. *Eur Radiol* 2006; 16: 256-268.

[39] Achenbach S, Ropers D, Kuettner A, et al. Contrast-enhanced coronary artery visualization by dual-source computed tomography-initial experience. *Eur J Radiol* 2006; 57: 331-335.

[40] Yoshimura N, Sabir A, Kubo T, et al. Correlation between image noise and body weight in coronary CTA with 16-row MDCT. *Acad Radiol* 2006; 13: 324-328.

[41] Das M, Mahnken AH, Muhlenbruch G, et al. Individually adapted examination protocols for reduction of radiation exposure for 16-MDCT chest examinations. *AJR Am J Roentgenol* 2005; 184: 1437-1443.

Chapter 5

Dual-Source Coronary CT Angiography in Coronary Artery Disease: A Systematic Review of Diagnostic Value, Image Quality and Radiation Dose

Abstract

To perform a systematic review of the diagnostic value, image quality and radiation dose of dual-source CT (DSCT) coronary angiography in the diagnosis of coronary artery disease (CAD) when compared to invasive coronary angiography. A search of four databases was performed to identify studies investigating the diagnostic value of DSCT coronary angiography in the diagnosis of coronary artery disease. Diagnostic value of DSCT coronary angiography was compared to invasive coronary angiography and analyzed at patient-based, vessel- and segment-based analysis. Twenty-nine studies met selection criteria and were included for analysis. Pooled estimates and 95% confidence interval (CI) of sensitivity, specificity, positive predictive value and negative predictive value of DSCT coronary angiography were 98% (95% CI: 99%, 99%), 83% (95% CI: 79%, 86%), 88% (95% CI: 86%, 91%), and 97% (95% CI: 95%, 99%), at patient-based analysis. The mean values of sensitivity, specificity, positive predictive value and negative predictive value of DSCT coronary angiography were 92% (95% CI: 89%, 95%), 90% (95% CI: 85%, 95%), 77% (95% CI: 71%, 83%) and 97% (95% CI: 96%, 98%), at vessel-based analysis; 89% (95% CI: 85%, 93%), 94% (95% CI: 92%, 96%), 76% (95% CI: 70%, 81%) and 98% (95% CI: 97%, 99%), at segment-based analysis, respectively. The mean effective dose of DSCT coronary angiography was 12.3 mSv (95% CI: 10.6, 14 mSv). Diagnostic performance of DSCT coronary angiography was independent of variable heart rates. The main factor that affects the diagnostic value of DSCT coronary angiography is presence of severe calcification, since high coronary calcium scores (>400) resulted in significant decrease of specificity and positive predictive value ($p<0.05$). DSCT coronary angiography has high diagnostic accuracy in the assessment of coronary artery disease, and its diagnostic performance remains high in the presence of high heart rates.

Keywords: Coronary CT angiography, dual-source CT, diagnostic value, image quality, radiation dose

5.1. Introduction

The advent of multislice CT technology has led to an increasing use of the modality in the diagnosis of coronary artery disease (CAD) [1-4]. With increased spatial and temporal resolution, diagnostic image quality and accuracy of coronary CT angiography has considerably improved. Studies using coronary CT angiography with 64-slice technology have reported a high diagnostic accuracy for the diagnosis of CAD [5-10]. In particular the high negative predictive value of more than 95% has indicated the reliability of 64-slice coronary CT angiography to exclude CAD [8-10]. Despite these promising results with 64-slice CT, diagnostic accuracy of 64-slice coronary CT angiography was reported to be affected by high heart rates and severe coronary calcifications [6, 8, 11, 12].

Dual-source CT (DSCT, Siemens, Germany) represents the recently developed multislice CT scanner, which enables a high temporal resolution of 83 ms in a single-segment reconstruction mode through simultaneous acquisition of cardiac images with two X-ray tubes and detectors [13]. The increased temporal resolution of the DSCT scanner makes cardiac imaging less dependent on a patient's heart rate. Since its introduction in 2005, DSCT coronary angiography has been illustrated to show improvements in the image quality and diagnostic accuracy in the diagnosis of coronary artery stenosis [14-20]. However, the reported diagnostic value of DSCT coronary angiography is variable, with wide ranges of diagnostic performance from patient-based to vessel-based and segment-based analysis [21]. Thus, the questions have to be addressed, which are: Does DSCT coronary angiography have adequate diagnostic value to be used as an alternative to invasive coronary angiography and is DSCT coronary angiography not influenced by heart rate or other factors? The aim of this chapter is to conduct a systematic review of the diagnostic value of DSCT coronary angiography in the diagnosis of CAD, according to the currently published studies.

5.2. Materials and Methods

5.2.1. Data Selection and Literature Searching

The literature search for relevant references was performed using different databases including Pubmed/Medline, ScienceDirect, Scopus and Embase to cover studies describing the diagnostic value of dual-source 64-slice coronary CT angiography in CAD between 2006 (DSCT was first introduced in 2006) and 2012 (last search was done in July 2012). The terms used for identification of references were‘ dual-source slice CT and coronary artery disease/stenosis’, ‘dual-source coronary CT angiography’, ‘dual-source CT angiography in CAD’ and ‘dual-source 64-slice CT in CAD’. The search was limited to include all the studies that have been published in the English language and were on human subjects. Case reports, conference abstracts, review articles, in vitro studies and articles investigating the coronary stent or bypass graft treatments were excluded from the analysis. In addition, the reference lists of identified articles were checked to obtain additional relevant articles.

Studies were included in the systematic review if they met all of the following criteria: (a) patients must be adults with suspected or known CAD who underwent both DSCT coronary angiography (first generation DSCT scanner) with use of retrospective ECG-gating, as studies performed with prospective ECG-triggering were discussed in Chapter 10; (b) studies included at least 10 patients; (c) assessment or comparison of DSCT coronary angiography with invasive coronary angiography was focused on the visualization of coronary arteries and detection or exclusion of CAD; (d) diagnostic value of DSCT coronary angiography was clearly stated and addressed (lumen stenosis >50% as significant stenosis) when compared to invasive coronary angiography in terms of sensitivity, specificity, positive predictive value (PPV), negative predictive value (NPV), either according to patients-based, vessel-based or segments-based assessment.

5.2.2. Data Extraction

Data were extracted repeatedly based on study design and procedure techniques. The reviewer looked for the following characteristics in each study: year of publication; number of patients included in each study; mean age; mean heart rate; number of male patients; mean body mass index (BMI); number of patients receiving β–blockers; prevalence of suspected or known CAD; assessable coronary segments in each study; image quality assessment (qualitative or quantitative analysis); coronary artery calcium scores; radiation dose associated with DSCT coronary angiography; diagnostic accuracy of DSCT coronary angiography when compared to invasive coronary angiography in terms of the sensitivity, specificity, PPV, NPV and main factors affecting the visualization of coronary arteries or diagnostic performance. All diagnostic accuracy estimates referred to segment/vessel/patient-based assessment.

A formal consensus method, QUADAS" (Quality Assessment of Diagnostic Accuracy Studies) was performed by one author for the quality assessment of diagnostic accuracy in these studies. The QUADAS is regarded as an important tool for quality assessment in systematic reviews as it enables to develop and evaluate an evidence-based quality of individual studies in terms of potential for bias, lack of applicability and quality of reporting [22].

5.2.3. Image Quality Assessment

Quantitative and qualitative assessments of diagnostic image quality recorded in each study were analysed. Quantitative image quality was determined by measuring signal-to-noise ratio (SNR) and contrast-to-noise ratio (CNR) for comparisons among the studies. SNR was calculated as the mean Hounsfield unit (HU) of particular region of interest (ROI) divided by image noise. CNR was defined as the difference of attenuation values of the contrast enhancement at two different regions (eg. left ventricular chamber and left ventricular wall) and then divided by image noise. Image noise is a standard deviation, SD of HU measured at selected anatomical regions.

Qualitative assessment of image quality was carried out on a per-segment basis by using of three- to five-point Likert ranking scale. The coronary segments were analyzed and the results were documented and categorized as percentage of assessable and non-assessable coronary segments. The coronary arteries were characterized into 13-17 segments according to the classification by American Heart Association (AHA) [23] and the extent of stenosis was evaluated in each segment with more than 50% coronary stenosis being defined as significant.

5.2.4. Statistical Analysis

All of the data was entered into SPSS (version 19.0) for analysis. Sensitivity, specificity, PPV and NPV estimates for each study were independently combined across studies using a fixed effects model. Between-study heterogeneity of the sensitivity, specificity, PPV and NPV estimates was tested using the Mantel-Haenszel Chi-squared test with n-1 degree of freedom (n is the number of studies). Pooled sensitivity, specificity, PPV and NPV values on patient-based assessment were entered into Meta Disc (V 1.4, Meta Analysis for Diagnostic and Screening Trials) for analysis, while the mean values of sensitivity, specificity, PPV and NPV values on vessel-based and segment-based assessment were analysed using SPSS. Statistical hypotheses (2-tailed) were tested at the 5% level of significance.

5.3. Results

Figure 5.1 is the flow chart showing studies that were obtained through the review process. After searching through these databases, 3407 articles were identified, of which 52 potentially relevant articles were selected for full-text assessment. Twenty-nine studies met our selection criteria, while the remaining 23 studies were excluded due to various reasons: coronary CT angiography performed with high-pitch protocol (n=14) and with prospective ECG-triggering (n=4); contents duplicates (n=3); results not presented to enable statistical analysis of diagnostic accuracy (n=2).

5.3.1. Study Characteristics

The characteristics of the eligible studies [17-19, 24-49] are presented in Table 5.1. The 29 studies enrolled 2648 patients (median, 75 patients, range, 15-436 patients). The mean age of the patients ranged from 58 to 71 years (median, 63 years). Of 29 studies, all were performed on dual-source 64-slice Siemens CT scanners (Somatom Definition, Siemens Medical Solutions, Forchheim, Germany) with temporal resolution of 83 ms. All of the coronary CT angiography was performed with retrospectively ECG-gated scans, while the studies performed with prospectively ECG-triggering or with high pitch protocols were discussed in Chapter 10.

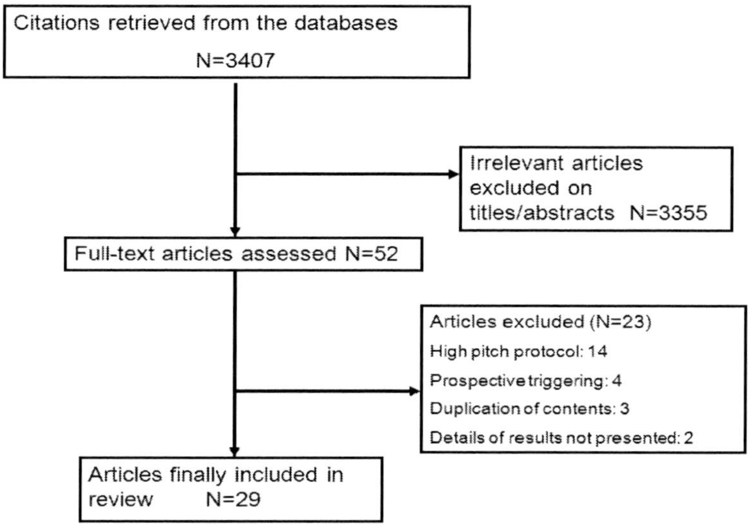

Figure 5.1. Flow chart shows the search strategy to obtain eligible references on dual-source coronary CT angiography.

It was found that the male patients were most commonly affected with CAD, with the mean value of 69% (range, 43% to 85%). The mean heart rate of patients during CT scan ranged from 59 to 89 beats per minute (bpm) across studies (median, 68 bpm). Beta-blocker was only used in 4 studies, and no heart rate control was implemented in 22 studies, while in the remaining study, information about beta-blocker usage was not available. The percentage of assessable segments was available in 24 studies with the mean value and 95% CI being 97% (96%, 98%). Coronary artery calcium scores were reported in 7 studies with the mean value and 95% CI being 690 (519, 862).

5.3.2. Radiation Dose

Information about radiation dose was available in 17 studies, while in the remaining studies, this was not reported. The estimated mean effective dose and 95% CI was 12.3 mSv (95% CI: 10.6, 14 mSv), and it ranged from 5.8 to 18.4 mSv with retrospectively ECG-gated scans. ECG-controlled tube current modulation was the most common approach used in these studies for dose reduction, while a tube voltage of 120 kVp was applied across all studies, except in two studies, in which 100 kVp was applied in patients with BMI less than 30 kg/m^2 [34, 35].

5.3.3. Coronary Segments Included in the Analysis

Although the AHA classification system was used in all of the 29 studies, different coronary segments were included for analysis among these studies. A 17-segment AHA system was used in 5 studies, followed by 16-segment method in 4 studies, 15-segment method in 8 studies, and 13-segment method in 6 studies. Details of the coronary segments were not available in the remaining 6 studies.

Table 5.1. Study characteristics of dual-source coronary CT angiography in coronary artery disease

Studies	Year of publication	Detector collimation	No. Patients	No. of cases β blocker %	Mean age (yrs)	No. of Male	HR	BMI	Assessable segments (%)	Calcium score	Effective dose (mSv)
Achenbach et al [a] (17)	2008	2x32x0.6	53	0	61±11	35	69±14	NA	96	NA	14.5±3.3
Achenbach et al [b] (17)	2008	2x32x0.6	47	92	63±11	29	59±10	NA	97	NA	14.8±3.5
Alkadhi et al (18)	2008	2x32x0.6	150	0	62.9±12.1	103	68.5±12.6	26.5±4.2	98.1	309±408	7-9
Brodoefel et al [a] (19)	2008	2x32x0.6	125	0	64	85	63±13.1/ 64.2±13.1/ 65.7±12.1	28.4±4.1	91.8	491±689/ 732±927/ 741±968	NA
Brodoefel et al [b] (24)	2008	2x32x0.6	100	0	62±10	80	64.9±13.2	NA	98.4	786.5±965.9	NA
Burgstahler et al (25)	2007	2x32x0.6	41	85	66.2±8.4	35	64±14	28±4.4	90.2	1391±966	NA
Chen et al (26)	2010	2x32x0.6	110	0	60.7	68	86.4	NA	98.6	NA	NA
Fang et al (27)	2010	2x32x0.6	89	0	59.6	57	88	NA	98.8	NA	11.2-18.5 (depending on HR)
Heuschmid et al (28)	2007	2x32x0.6	51	0	64±10	37	65±14	28± 4	100	779±996	NA
Johnson et al (29)	2007	2x32x0.6	35	0	60±12	24	NA	NA	98	NA	4.6-7.5
Leber et al (30)	2007	2x32x0.6	90	0	58±8	57	73	NA	98.7	NA	9.6 (7.1-12.3)
Leschka et al (31)	2008	2x32x0.6	74	0	61.7±12.3	50	67.7±13.3	27.2±4	97.9	720±968	7-9
Lin et al (32)	2010	2x32x0.6	44	0	61.2±10	34	66.9±14.2	26±2.7	NA	NA	NA
Marvan et al [a] (33)	2010	2x32x0.6	60	53	71±7	34	70±15	29±5	NA	NA	16±5
Marvan et al [b] (34)	2011	2x32x0.6	88	NA	66±11	38	61±9	27±5	NA	364	7±5
Meng et al (35)	2009	2x32x0.6	109	0	63±9	68	71.8±13.2	26.9±3.3	98	821±904	NA
Moon et al (36)	2011	2x32x0.6	131	78	64.5±8.9	85	58.9±8	NA	97	NA	5.8±2 (5.5±1.9/ 6.7±2.2)
Oncel at al (37)	2007	2x32x0.6	15	0	58.5±9	9	83.7±8.9	±	94	NA	13.8±1.37
Piers et al (38)	2008	2x32x0.6	60	NA	64 (57-70)	51	63±12	NA	93	NA	7.3
Rist et al (39)	2009	2x32x0.6	68	0	64±11	54	77±25	NA	92	NA	13.28
Rixe et al (40)	2009	2x32x0.6	76	0	65±10	47	68±9	28.7±4.8	100	337±560	13.8±6.7/ 14.3±5.6*

Studies	Year of publication	Detector collimation	No. Patients	No. of cases β blocker %	Mean age (yrs)	No. of Male	HR	BMI	Assessable segments (%)	Calcium score	Effective dose (mSv)
Ropers et al (41)	2007	2x32x0.6	100	0	61	63	64±13	28	96	NA	15.3±3.7/ 15.9±3.1 (<65bpm vs>65bpm)
Scheffel et al (42)	2006	2x32x0.6	30	0	63.1±11.3	24	70.3±14.2	28.3±3.9	98.6	821±904	NA
Tsiflikas et al [a] (43)	2010	2x32x0.6	170	0	64±9	124	64±12	28±4	100	686±976	NA
Tsiflikas et al [b] (44)	2010	2x32x0.6	44	0	68±9	31	69±14	27.9±4.3	95	NA	NA
Weustink et al[a] (45)	2007	2x32x0.6	100	0	61±11	79	68±11	NA	100	NA	11.1-14.4: low HR<56, 10.7-13.8. HR 68 8.3-9.6, HR 81
Weustink et al[b] (46)	2009	2x32x0.6	436	0	61.6±10.6	301	69.8±23.9/ 68.8±22.7	NA	NA	NA	10.7±3.6/14.2± 3.2/18.4±3.5
Xu et al (47)	2010	2x32x0.6	84	0	64.6	58	71.4±11.4	NA	100	NA	16.1±3.1
Yang et al (48)	2010	2x32x0.6	46	0	65±5.7	36	NA	NA	NA	NA	NA
Zhang et al (49)	2011	2x32x0.6	22	0	72.1±8.3	14	89±13	22.5±3.7	97	NA	8.7±4.6

Achenbach et al (a) and (b) compared two groups of patients, with no heart rate control and heart rate control subgroups.

Brodoefel et al (a) compared the effect of different BMI ranges on diagnostic value, while Brodoefel et al (b) focused on the effect of variable heart rates.

Rixe et al. * for patients with HR >70 bpm

Tsiflikas et al (b) and Marvan et al (a): patients with atrial fibrillation were included in the study. Marvan et al (b): patients with uncontrolled hypertension were included.

Weustink et al (b): standard protocol vs ECG pulsing protocol.

HR-heart rate, NA-not available.

Table 5.2. Quality assessment (QUADAS)

Study	Item 1	Item 2	Item 3	Item 4	Item 5	Item 6	Item 7	Item 8	Item 9	Item 10	Item 11	Item 12	Item 13	Item 14
Achenbach et al (17)	Yes	Yes	Yes	Yes	Yes	Yes	Yes	Yes	Yes	Yes	Yes	Yes	Yes	Yes
Achenbach et al (17)	Yes	Yes	Yes	Yes	Yes	Yes	Yes	Yes	Yes	Yes	Yes	Yes	Yes	Yes
Alkadhi et al (18)	Yes	Yes	Yes	Yes	Yes	Yes	Yes	Yes	Yes	Yes	Yes	Yes	Yes	Yes
Brodoefel et al [a] (19)	Yes	Yes	Yes	Yes	Yes	Yes	Yes	Yes	Yes	Yes	Yes	Yes	Yes	Yes
Brodoefel et al [b] (24)	Yes	Yes	Yes	Yes	Yes	Yes	Yes	Yes	Yes	Yes	Yes	Yes	Yes	Yes
Burgstahler et al (25)	Yes	Yes	Yes	Yes	Yes	Yes	Yes	Yes	Yes	Yes	Yes	Yes	Yes	Yes
Chen et al (26)	Yes	Yes	Yes	Yes	Yes	Yes	Yes	Yes	Yes	Yes	Yes	Yes	Yes	NA
Fang et al (27)	Yes	Yes	Yes	Yes	Yes	Yes	Yes	Yes	Yes	Yes	Yes	Yes	Yes	NA
Heuschmid et al (28)	Yes	Yes	Yes	Yes	Yes	Yes	Yes	Yes	Yes	Yes	Yes	Yes	Yes	Yes
Johnson et al (29)	Yes	Yes	Yes	Yes	Yes	Yes	Yes	Yes	Yes	Yes	Yes	Yes	Yes	Yes
Leber et al (30)	Yes	Yes	Yes	Yes	Yes	Yes	Yes	Yes	Yes	Yes	Unclear	Yes	Yes	Yes
Leschka et al (31)	Yes	Yes	Yes	Yes	Yes	Yes	Yes	Yes	Unclear	Yes	Yes	Yes	Yes	Yes
Lin et al (32)	Yes	Yes	Yes	Yes	Yes	Yes	Yes	Yes	Yes	Yes	Yes	Yes	Yes	Yes
Marvan et al [a] (33)	Yes	Yes	Yes	Yes	Yes	Yes	Yes	Yes	Yes	Yes	Yes	Yes	Yes	Yes
Marvan et al [b] (34)	Yes	Yes	Yes	Yes	Yes	Yes	Yes	Yes	Yes	Yes	Yes	Yes	Yes	Yes
Meng et al (35)	Yes	Yes	Yes	Yes	Yes	Yes	Yes	Yes	Yes	Yes	Yes	Yes	Yes	NA
Moon et al (36)	Yes	Yes	Yes	Yes	Yes	Yes	Yes	Yes	Yes	Yes	Yes	Yes	Yes	NA
Oncel at al (37)	Yes	Yes	Yes	Yes	Yes	Yes	Yes	Yes	Yes	Yes	Yes	Yes	Yes	NA
Piers et al (38)	Yes	Yes	Yes	Yes	Yes	Yes	Yes	Yes	Yes	Yes	Yes	Yes	Yes	Yes
Rist et al (39)	Yes	Yes	Yes	Yes	Yes	Yes	Yes	Yes	Yes	Yes	Yes	Yes	Yes	Yes
Rixe et al (40)	Yes	Yes	Yes	Yes	Yes	Yes	Yes	Yes	Yes	Yes	Yes	Yes	Yes	NA
Ropers et al (41)	Yes	Yes	Yes	Yes	Yes	Yes	Yes	Yes	Yes	Yes	Yes	Yes	Yes	NA

Study	Item 1	Item 2	Item 3	Item 4	Item 5	Item 6	Item 7	Item 8	Item 9	Item 10	Item 11	Item 12	Item 13	Item 14
Scheffel et al (42)	Yes	Yes	Yes	Yes	Yes	Yes	Yes	Yes	Yes	Yes	Yes	Yes	Yes	NA
Tsiflikas et al [a] (43)	Yes	Yes	Yes	Yes	Yes	Yes	Yes	Yes	Yes	Yes	Yes	Yes	Yes	NA
Tsiflikas et al [b] (44)	Yes	Yes	Yes	Yes	Yes	Yes	Yes	Yes	Yes	Yes	Yes	Yes	Yes	NA
Weustink et al[a] (45)	Yes	Yes	Yes	Yes	Yes	Yes	Yes	Yes	Yes	Yes	Yes	Yes	Yes	Yes
Weustink et al[b] (46)	Yes	Yes	Yes	Yes	Yes	Yes	Yes	Yes	Yes	Yes	Yes	Yes	Yes	Yes
Xu et al (47)	Yes	No	Yes	Yes	Yes	Yes	Yes	Yes	Yes	Yes	Yes	Yes	Unclear	NA
Yang et al (48)	Yes	Yes	Yes	Yes	Yes	Yes	Yes	Yes	Yes	Yes	Yes	Yes	Unclear	Yes
Zhang et al (49)	Yes	Yes	Yes	Yes	Yes	Yes	Yes	Yes	Yes	Yes	Yes	Yes	Yes	NA

Item 1: was the spectrum of patients representative of the patients who will receive the test in practice?
Item 2: were selection criteria clearly described?
Item 3: is the reference standard likely to correctly classify the target condition?
Item 4: is the time period between reference and standard and index test short enough to be reasonably sure that the target condition did not change between the two tests?
Item 5: did the whole sample or a random selection of the sample, receive verification using a reference standard of diagnosis?
Item 6: did patients receive the same reference standard regardless of the index test results?
Item 7: was the reference standard independent of the index test (i.e., the index test did not form part of the reference standard)?
Item 8: was the execution of the index test described in the sufficient detail to permit replication of the test?
Item 9: was the execution of the reference standard described in the sufficient detail to permit its replication?
Item 10: were the index test results interpreted without knowledge of the results of the reference standard?
Item 11: were the reference standard results interpreted without knowledge of the results of the index test?
Item 12: were the same clinical data available when test results were interpreted as would be available when the test is used in practice?
Item 13: were uninterpretable/intermediate test results reported?
Item 14: were withdrawals from the study explained?
NA-not available.

5.3.4. Image Quality Assessment

Subjective assessment of DSCT coronary angiography images was conducted in 24 studies by two observers who were blinded to the results of invasive coronary angiography, with use of 2- to 5-point scoring scale applied in 14 studies. Only one observer was involved in the evaluation of image quality in 4 studies, while in the remaining study, details of the observer assessment were not available. In contrast, in more than half of the studies (69%), invasive coronary angiographic images were evaluated only by one observer, while in 8 studies two observers were involved in the assessment of angiographic images, and in the remaining study, the information was not available. Quantitative assessment of image quality was only conducted in one study [35] with use of contrast-to-noise ratio to determine the image quality.

Quality assessment of all included studies based on the updated QUADAS is shown in Table 5.2. Overall, the study quality was satisfactory. Of all 29 studies, the investigators clearly explained that readers interpreted DSCT coronary angiography results without any knowledge of the invasive coronary angiography results and vice versa. In addition, operators and readers of DSCT coronary angiography were unaware of patient history and symptoms in all studies.

5.3.5. Diagnostic Value of DSCT Coronary Angiography: Patient-Based Analysis

Of 29 studies, evaluation of DSCT coronary angiography in CAD at patient-based assessment was available in 16 studies with 36 comparisons. No statistical heterogeneity in sensitivity was found for these analyses according to patient-based assessment, however, significant difference in specificity was found among these studies ($p=0.001$). The pooled estimates across studies were used to demonstrate the diagnostic performance. Pooled estimates and 95% CI of the sensitivity, specificity, PPV and NPV of DSCT coronary angiography were 98% (95% CI: 99%, 99%), 83% (95% CI: 79%, 86%), 88% (95% CI: 86%, 91%), and 97% (95% CI: 95%, 99%) (Figs 5.2, 5.3).

Eight out of 16 studies involved multiple comparisons, with 6 studies comparing different heart rates with regard to the diagnostic value of DSCT coronary angiography [17, 18, 30, 32, 35, 42]. The mean sensitivity, specificity, PPV and NPV and 95% CI were 96% (95% CI: 93%. 99%), 77% (95% CI: 60%, 94%), 84% (95% CI: 74%, 94%) and 93% (95% CI: 79%, 100%) for patients with heart rate less than 65 bpm; 98% (95% CI: 95%, 100%), 79% (95% CI: 60%, 98%), 83% (95% CI: 74%, 92%) and 99% (95% CI: 96%, 100%) for patients with heart rate greater than 65 bpm. There was no statistically significant difference in the diagnostic performance between these two groups ($p>0.05$).

One study compared the effect of different BMI and calcium score values on diagnostic performance [18], with no significant change observed in patients with BMI >26 kg/m^2. In the presence of moderate and high calcium scores, the sensitivity was decreased compared to the corresponding lower calcium score group, although no significant change was observed in the sensitivity, PPV and NPV [18]. Another study compared DSCT coronary angiography to the protocol of combining calcium score with coronary CT angiography [31], with combined method showing improvement in the specificity in patients with non-evaluable coronary segments. The remaining study compared standard coronary CT angiography (non-pulsing protocol) with optimal ECG pulsing protocol [46], with significant reduction in radiation dose while preserving the diagnostic performance of DSCT coronary angiography.

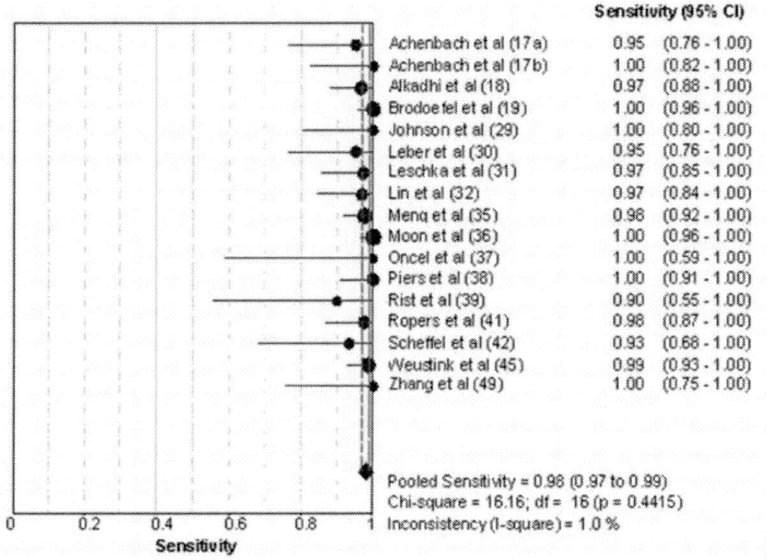

Figure 5.2. Plot of pooled sensitivity of dual-source coronary CT angiography compared to invasive coronary angiography in 16 studies based on patient-based assessment. CI-confidence interval.

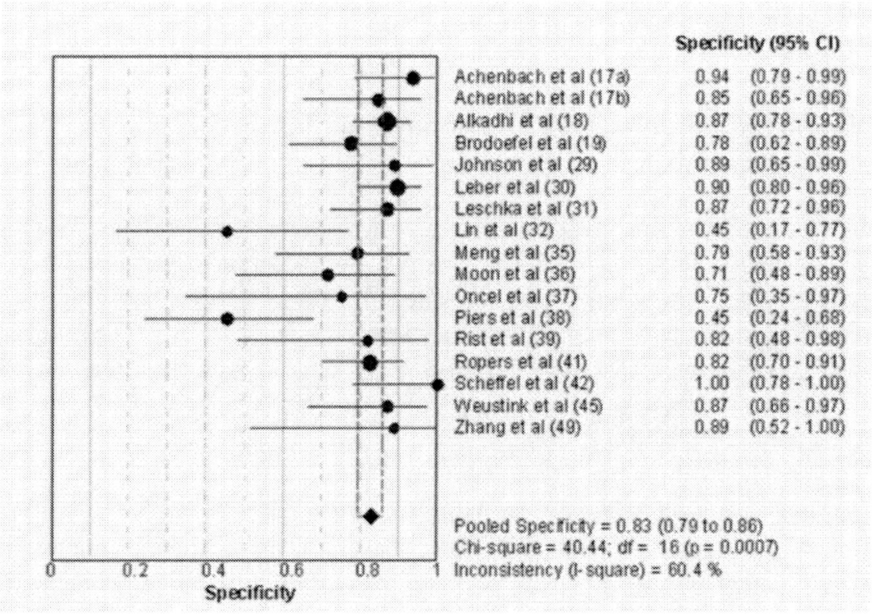

Figure 5.3. Plot of pooled specificity of dual-source coronary angiography compared to invasive coronary angiography in 16 studies based on patient-based assessment. Note that there are two studies [32, 38] reporting very low specificity (<50%), thus, this contributes to the relatively low pooled specificity. CI-confidence interval.

5.3.6. Diagnostic Value of DSCT Coronary Angiography: Vessel-Based Analysis

Of 29 studies, evaluation of DSCT coronary angiography in CAD at vessel-based assessment was available in 13 studies with 23 comparisons, as four studies involved multiple comparisons.

Severe heterogeneity/inconsistency was noticed at the vessel-based and segment-based assessment levels ($p<0.05$), so pooling was avoided, and only the mean values across these studies were described. The mean values of sensitivity, specificity, PPV and NPV and 95% CI were 92% (95% CI: 89%, 95%), 90% (95% CI: 85%, 95%), 77% (95% CI: 71%, 83%) and 97% (95% CI: 96%, 98%), according to vessel-based assessment.

Four out of 13 studies involved comparison of the effect of different heart rates on the diagnostic performance of DSCT coronary angiography in the diagnosis of CAD, and analysis showed there was no significant difference between two groups (patients with heart rate less than 65 bpm versus patients with heart rate greater than 65 bpm) ($p>0.05$).

The mean values of sensitivity, specificity, PPV and NPV and 95% CI were 95% (95% CI: 87%, 100%), 92% (95% CI: 85%, 98%), 81% (95% CI: 66%, 95%) and 98% (95% CI: 97%, 99%) for patients with heart rate less than 65 bpm; 94% (95% CI: 92%,. 96%), 89% (95% CI: 72%, 100%), 80% (95% CI: 65%, 95%) and 98% (95% CI: 96%, 99%) for patients with heart rate greater than 65 bpm.

One study compared the effect of different coronary calcium scores on the diagnostic performance [31], and DSCT coronary angiography showed high diagnostic accuracy in patients with coronary calcification. Specificity and PPV was significantly reduced in the presence of severe calcification (coronary calcium score >400).

5.3.7. Diagnostic Value of DSCT Coronary Angiography: Segment-Based Analysis

Evaluation of DSCT coronary angiography in CAD at segment-based analysis was available in 24 studies with 63 comparisons. As mentioned in the section of 5.3.3, different numbers of coronary segments were included in these studies, resulting in severe heterogeneity/inconsistency at the segment-based assessment levels ($p<0.05$), thus, only the mean values across these studies were described. The mean sensitivity, specificity, PPV and NPV and 95% CI was 89% (95% CI: 85%, 93%), 94% (95% CI: 92%, 96%), 76% (95% CI: 70%, 81%) and 98% (95% CI: 97%, 99%).

5.3.7.1. Effect of Heart Rate on Diagnostic Value

Ten studies compared the effect of different heart rates on the diagnostic performance of DSCT coronary angiography in CAD, with no significant difference found between the patients with heart rate less than 65 bpm and those with greater than 65 bpm ($p>0.05$). The mean value of sensitivity, specificity, PPV and NPV is shown in Table 5.3.

Table 5.3. Mean values of sensitivity, specificity, PPV and NPV of dual-source coronary CT angiography according to segment-based assessment

Factors to be assessed		Sensitivity (95% CI)	Specificity (95% CI)	Positive predictive value (95% CI)	Negative predictive value (95% CI)
Heart rates	<65 bpm	93% (90%, 95%)	95% (93%, 98%)	78% (71%, 84%)	99% (98%, 99%)
	>65 bpm	93% (91%, 94%)	96% (93%, 99%)	79% (72%, 85%)	99% (98%, 99%)
Coronary calcium scores	Low CAC	89% (82%, 96%)	97% (95%, 100%)	75% (57%, 91%)	99% (99%, 100%)
	Moderate CAC	94% (85%, 100%)	95% (91%, 99%)	77% (69%, 84%)	99% (97%, 100%)
	High CAC	96% (92%, 99%)	87% (76%, 97%)	71% (50%, 92%)	98% (96%, 100%)
Body mass index	<25 kg/m^2	93% (74%, 99%)	96% (90%, 99%)	73% (71%, 76%)	99% (94%, 100%)
	>25 kg/m^2	93% (55%, 99%)	94% (69%, 100%)	77% (73%, 83%)	99% (91%, 100%)

bpm-beats per minute, CAC: coronary calcium score, CI-confidence interval, PPV-positive predictive value, NPV-negative predictive value.

5.3.7.2. Effect of Coronary Calcium Score on Diagnostic Value

Four studies provided coronary calcium scores and their corresponding effects on diagnostic performance of DSCT coronary angiography. Diagnostic specificity, PPV and NPV were decreased in patients with high calcium scores. Significant differences were found in specificity and NPV when comparing groups of low calcium scores with high calcium scores ($p<0.05$); however, no significant difference was found in the sensitivity when comparing groups with low calcium scores to those with moderate and high calcium scores ($p>0.05$). The mean diagnostic value corresponding to different calcium scores is presented in Table 5.3.3.

5.3.7.3. Effect of Body Mass Index on Diagnostic Value

Two studies compared the effect of BMI on the diagnostic performance of DSCT coronary angiography, and there was no significant difference between different BMI groups with regard to the diagnostic value. The mean value of sensitivity, specificity, PPV and NPV is shown in Table 5.3.3.

Discussion

This systematic review has three important findings which are considered valuable for clinical utilization of DSCT coronary angiography in the diagnosis of CAD. Firstly, DSCT coronary angiography has high diagnostic sensitivity (>90%) in the detection of CAD at per-patient, vessel- and segment-based analysis. The consistently high negative predictive value (mean 97%) is the most outstanding performance of this technique that indicates the reliability of a negative scan for exclusion of significant CAD. Secondly, diagnostic value of DSCT coronary angiography is independent of heart rate, thus, this technique can be extended to patients with high or irregular heart rate and in most cases no heart rate control is needed. Thirdly, diagnostic performance of DSCT coronary angiography is affected by high calcium scores, thus, in patients with extensive coronary calcification, image findings should be interpreted with caution due to high percentage of false positive cases.

Sixty-four slice CT shows improved image quality when compared to early generation of 4- and 16-slice scanners, owing to further technical improvements in scanning techniques, resulting particularly in improved temporal resolution [50]. Several systematic reviews and meta-analyses of studies on the use of 64-slice CT coronary angiography reported mean sensitivities and specificities ranging from 85% to 99%, and 86% to 96%, respectively [51-54]. However, its temporal and spatial resolutions are insufficient for precise assessment of coronary arteries, particularly in patients with uncontrolled heart rates. Thus, the use of beta-blockers to lower the heart rate to less than 65 bpm is frequently used in 64-slice CT imaging of patients with suspected CAD. The introduction of DSCT marked another technological improvement of coronary CT angiography in cardiac imaging, as the temporal resolution is further increased from 165 ms to 83 ms, thus eliminating the need to control the heart rate during the scan [55, 56].

Studies comparing DSCT with single-source CT demonstrated that DSCT maintains high diagnostic accuracy in the diagnostic examination of a wide range of patients subsets, e.g. patients with higher and even irregular heart rates (including atrial fibrillation) [55, 56]. Despite slightly lower per-segment evaluability in patients with higher heart rates, DSCT did not show decrease in diagnostic accuracy for the detection of coronary stenoses [30, 41]. This analysis is consistent with these reports, as the assessable segment by DSCT coronary angiography is 97%, and the diagnostic accuracy remains high in the presence of high heart rates, according to per-patient, per-vessel and per-segment analysis. DSCT improves temporal resolution which is vital in those patients who cannot have beta blockade. Therefore, this may result in less strict criteria for application of DSCT coronary angiography in routine clinical circumstances in which there are contraindications to beta-blocker.

In this systematic review, 14% of the patients among 29 studies received beta-blocker before coronary CT angiography examination. Although this is slightly higher than the 8% of the total number of patients receiving beta-blocker reported by Salavati et al [57], it is much lower than the 41%-76% of patients that received beta-blocker undergoing 64-slice coronary CT angiography [52, 54]. Although the range of mean heart rates (59-89 bpm) in the studies performed by DSCT is similar to that reported by Salavati et al [57], which is between 56-86 bpm, the median values in this analysis (68 bpm) are higher than the previous analysis (64 bpm). Despite the relatively high mean heart rates in these patients, the diagnostic accuracy of DSCT coronary angiography in this analysis aligns with previous meta-analyses [21, 57], indicating the improved diagnostic performance of DSCT coronary angiography.

The diagnostic value of coronary CT angiography is widely known to be affected by the heavy calcification in the coronary artery tree. High-density calcification produces blooming artefacts which lead to overestimation of the degree of coronary stenosis, thus resulting in low positive predictive value and specificity. This is confirmed in this analysis, as a significant decrease in specificity was found in patients with high calcium scores (more than 400) when compared to patients with low or moderate calcium scores. This is confirmed by a recently published ACCURACY prospective multicentre study, which included patients with high calcium scores [58]. Patient-based specificity of 83% was reported in detecting significant coronary stenosis. In contrast, another study which excluded patients with a calcium score of more than 600, reported a specificity of 90% [59]. These conflicting findings represent the limitations of the current research results in the literature due to different study designs used in each single centre and the degree of strictness applied in controlling bias in the study. It has been shown that significant statistical heterogeneity exists among published studies, with smaller studies reporting higher diagnostic accuracy of coronary CT angiography in CAD [60]. Therefore, reports of the diagnostic value of DSCT coronary angiography in CAD in the literature need to be interpreted with caution.

The relatively high radiation dose associated with coronary CT angiography is a main source of concern [61]. With single-source 64-slice CT, improved temporal resolution is accompanied by increased radiation exposure to patients because faster gantry rotation requires a lower pitch (0.2-0.4) to acquire gapless cardiac images in the volume data coverage [62]. In patients with higher heart rate, pitch cannot be increased significantly due to multisegment reconstruction requiring a slow table speed to compensate for motion artefacts [63]. In contrast, with DSCT, the pitch value can be adapted to the heart rate, thus, multisegment reconstruction is not required, thereby limiting radiation dose with increased heart rate [27, 63]. The mean effective dose in this analysis is 12.3 mSv, which is similar to 11.2 mSv in patients with heart rate greater than 100 bpm in a previous report when compared to the high radiation dose of 18.5 mSv in the lower heart rate group [27]. ECG-controlled tube current modulation is the most common approach used for dose reduction which has been reported to reduce the effective dose by 50% [64, 65]. This is also widely used in the studies included in this analysis. Reduction of tube voltage from the routine 120 kVp to 100 or 80 kVp is also an effective approach for dose reduction, and this is recommended in patients with BMI less than 25 kg/m^2 [66-68]. Another dose-saving strategy is prospective ECG-triggering or step-and-shoot method. Coronary CT angiography using prospective ECG-triggering has been reported to significantly reduce radiation dose, with effective dose ranging from 2.7 mSv to 4.5 mSv [69-71]. Diagnostic value of prospectively ECG-triggered coronary CT angiography will be discussed in Chapters 9 and 10.

Some limitations in this systematic review should be addressed. Firstly, publication bias may have affected the results since we just included articles in English and excluded non-English references. Secondly, different groups, including patients with suspected CAD, known cases of CAD, or a mixture of both were enrolled among these studies, thus patient selection bias could potentially lead to overestimation of the diagnostic ability of DSCT coronary angiography to detect coronary stenosis. Thirdly, different segmentation models were used (range, 13-17 segments), as well as different reporting designs that might have influenced the absolute number of true and false interpretations in each study, consequently contributing to the biased pooled analysis. Lastly, the ideal subjects are patients with intermediate pretest probability of CAD [30], thus the performance of DSCT coronary angiography in an intermediate risk population need to be investigated.

In conclusion, this systematic review indicates that DSCT coronary angiography has high diagnostic accuracy in the diagnosis of coronary artery disease, even in the presence of high heart rates. Diagnostic performance of DSCT coronary angiography is affected by heavy calcification in the coronary arteries. DSCT coronary angiography is associated with high radiation dose, thus, further dose-reduction strategies need to be undertaken to reduce radiation exposure to patients while maintaining diagnostic image quality.

Acknowledgment

The author would like to thank Mr Gil Stevenson for his assistance in the statistical analysis of results.

References

[1] Wijns W. Diagnosis of coronary artery disease: In search of a ''One-Stop Shop''? *J Nucl Med* 2005;46: 904-5.

[2] Goldstein JA, Gallagher MJ, O'Neill WW, Ross MA, O'neil BJ, Raff GL. A randomized controlled trial of multi-slice coronary computed tomography for evaluation of acute chest pain. *J Am Coll Cardiol* 2007;49:863-871.

[3] Flohr TG, Schoepf UJ, Ohnsorge BM. Chasing the heart. New developments for cardiac CT. *J Thorac Imaging* 2007;22:4-16.

[4] Gasparovic H, Rybicki FJ, Millstine J, et al. Three dimensional computed tomographic imaging in planning the surgical approach for redo cardiac surgery after coronary revascularization. *Eur J Cardiothorac Surg* 2005;28:244-249.

[5] Leber AW, Knez A, von Ziegler F, et al. Quantification of obstructive and nonobstructive coronary lesions by 64-slice computed tomography: A comparative study with quantitative coronary angiography and intravascular ultrasound. *J Am Coll Cardiol* 2005; 46: 147-154.

[6] Leschka S, Alkadhi H, Plass A, et al. Accuracy of MSCT coronary angiography with 64-slice technology: first experience. *Eur Heart J* 2005, 26: 1482-1487.

[7] Plass A, Grunenfelder J, Leschka S, et al. Coronary artery imaging with 64-slice computed tomography from cardiac surgical perspective. *Eur J Radiol* 2006; 30: 109-116.

[8] Raff GL, Gallagher MJ, O'Neill WW, et al. Diagnostic accuracy of non-invasive coronary angiography using 64-slice spiral computed tomography. *J Am Coll Cardiol* 2005, 46: 552-557.

[9] Ehara M, Surmely JF, Kawai M, et al. Diagnostic accuracy of 64-slice computed tomography for detecting angiographically significant coronary artery stenosis in an unselected consecutive patient population: comparison with conventional invasive angiography. *Cir J* 2006; 70: 564-571.

[10] Nikolaou K, Knez A, Rist C, et al. Accuracy of 64-MDCT in the diagnosis of ischemic heart disease. *AJR Am J Roentgenol* 2006; 187: 111-117.

[11] Oncel D, Oncel G, Tastan A, Tamci B. Detection of significant coronary artery stenosis with 64-section MDCT angiography. *Eur J Radiol* 2007; 62: 394-405.

[12] Palumbo AA, Maffei E, Martini G, et cl. Coronary calcium score as gatekeeper for 64-slice computed tomography coronary angiography in patients with chest pain: per-segment and per-patient analysis. *Eur Radiol* 2009; 19: 2127-2135.

[13] Flohr TG, McCollough CH, Bruder H, et al. First performance evaluation of a dual-source CT (DSCT) system. *Eur Radiol* 2006; 16(2):256–268.

[14] Plass A, Azemaj N, Scheffel H, et al. Accuracy of dual-source computed tomography coronary angiography: evaluation with a standardised protocol for cardiac surgeons. *Eur J Cardiothorac Surg* 2009; 36(6):1011–1017.

[15] Alkadhi H, Stolzmann P, Desbiolles L, et al. Low-dose, 128-slice, dual-source CT coronary angiography: accuracy and radiation dose of the high-pitch and the step-and-shoot mode. *Heart* 2010; 96: 933-938.

[16] Donati QF, Scheffel H, Stolzmann P, et al. Combined cardiac CT and MRI for the comprehensive workup of hemodynamically relevant coronary stenoses. *AJR Am J Roentgenol* 2010; 914: 920-926.

[17] Achenbach S, Ropers D, Kuettner A, et al. Randomized comparison of 64-slice single- and dual-source computed tomography coronary angiography for the detection of coronary artery disease. *JACC Cardiovasc Imaging* 2008; 1: 177-86.

[18] Alkadhi H, Scheffel H, Desbiolles L, et al. Dual-source computed tomography coronary angiography: influence of obesity, calcium load, and heart rate on diagnostic accuracy. *Eur Heart J* 2008; 29: 766-776.

[19] Brodoefel H, Tsiflikas I, Burgstahler C, et al. Cardiac dual-source computed tomography: effect of body mass index on image quality and diagnostic accuracy. *Invest Radiol* 2008; 43: 712-718.

[20] Scheffel G, Alkadhi H, Leschka S, et al. Low-dose CT coronary angiography in the step-and-shoot mode: diagnostic performance. *Heart* 2008; 94: 1132-1137.

[21] Guo SL, Guo YM, Zhai YN, et al. Diagnostic accuracy of first generation dual-source computed tomography in the assessment of coronary artery disease: a meta-analysis from 24 studies. *Int J Cardiovasc Imaging* 2011; 27: 755-771.

[22] Whiting P, Rutjes AW, Reitsma JB, et al. The development of QUADAS: a tool for the quality assessment of studies of diagnostic accuracy included in systematic reviews. *BMC Med Res Methodol* 2003; 3:25.

[23] Austen WG, Edwards JE, Frye RL, et al. Report of the ad hoc committee for grading of coronary artery disease. A reporting system on patients evaluated for coronary artery disease. *Am Heart Assoc* 1975; 5-40.

[24] Brodoefel H, Burgstahler C, Tsiflikas I, et al. Dual-source CT: effect of heart rate, heart rate variability, and calcification on image quality and diagnostic accuracy. *Radiology* 2008; 247: 346-355.

[25] Burgstahler C, Reimann A, Drosch T, et al. Cardiac dual-source computed tomography in patients with severe coronary calcifications and a high prevalence of coronary artery disease. *J Cardiovasc Comput Tomogr* 2007; 1: 143-151.

[26] Chen H, Fang X, Hu X, et al. Efficacy of dual-source CT coronary angiography in evaluating coronary stenosis: initial experience. *Clin Imaging* 2010; 34: 165-171.

[27] Fang X, Chen H, Hu X, et al. Dual-source CT coronary angiography without heart rate or rhythm control in comparison with conventional coronary angiography. *Int J Cardiovasc Imaging* 2010; 26: 323-331.

[28] Heuschmid M, Burgstahler C, Reimann A, et al. Usefulness of noninvasive cardiac imaging using dual-source computed tomography in an unselected population with high prevalence of coronary artery disease. *Am J Cardiol* 2007; 100: 587-592.

[29] Johnson T, Nikolaou K, Busch S, et al. Diagnostic accuracy of dual-source computed tomography in the diagnosis of coronary artery disease. *Invest Radiol* 2007; 42: 684-691.

[30] Leber AW, Johnson T, Becker A, et al. Diagnostic accuracy of dual-source multi-slice CT coronary angiography in patients with an intermediate pretest likelihood for coronary artery disease. *Eur Heart J* 2007; 28 2354-2360.

[31] Leschka S, Scheffel H, Desbiolles L, et al. Combining dual-source computed tomography coronary angiography and calcium scoring: added value for the assessment of coronary artery disease. *Heart* 2008; 94: 1154-1161.

[32] Lin CJ, Hsu JC, Lai YJ, et al. Diagnostic accuracy of dual-source CT coronary angiography in a population unselected for degree of coronary artery calcification and without heart rate modification. *Clin Radiol* 2010; 65: 109-117.

[33] Marvan M, Pflederer T, Schepis T, et al. Accuracy of dual-source computed tomography to identify significant coronary artery disease in patients with atrial fibrillation: comparison with coronary angiography. *Eur Heart J* 2010; 31: 2230-2237.

[34] Marvan M, Pflederer T, Schepis T, et al. Accuracy of dual-source CT to identify significant coronary artery disease in patients with uncontrolled hypertension presenting with chest pain: comparison with coronary angiography. *Int J Cardiovasc Imaging* 2012; 28: 1173-1180.

[35] Meng L, Cui L, Cheng Y, et al. Effect of heart rate and coronary calcification on the diagnostic accuracy of the dual-source CT coronary angiography in patients with suspected coronary artery disease. *Korean J Radiol* 2009; 10: 347-354.

[36] Moon JH, Park EA, Lee W, et al. The diagnostic accuracy, image quality and radiation dose of 64-slice dual-source CT in daily practice: a single institution's experience. *Korean J Radiol* 2011; 12: 308-318.

[37] Oncel D, Oncel G, Tastan A. Effectiveness of dual-source CT coronary angiography for the evaluation of coronary artery disease in patients with atrial fibrillation: initial experience. *Radiology* 2007; 245: 703-711.

[38] Piers LH, Dikkers R, Willems TP, et al. Computed tomographic angiography or conventional coronary angiography in therapeutic decision-making. *Eur Heart J* 2008; 29: 2902-2907.

[39] Rist C, Johnson TR, Muller-Starck J, et al. Noninvasive coronary angiography using dual-source computed tomography in patients with atrial fibrillation. *Invest Radiol* 2009; 44: 159-167.

[40] Rixe J, Rolf A, Conradi G, et al. detection of relevant coronary artery disease using dual-source computed tomography in a high probability patient series: comparison with invasive angiography. *Circ J* 2009; 73: 316-322.

[41] Ropers U, Ropers D, Pflederer T, et al. Influence of heart rate on the diagnostic accuracy of dual-source computed tomography coronary angiography. *J Am Coll Cardiol* 2007; 50: 2393-2398.

[42] Scheffel H, Alkadhi H, Plass A, et al. Accuracy of dual-source CT coronary angiography: first experience in a high pre-test probability population without heart rate control. *Eur Radiol* 2006; 16: 2739-2747.

[43] Tsiflikas I, Brodoefel H, Reimann AJ, et al. Coronary CT angiography with dual source computed tomography in 170 patients. *Eur J Radiol* 2010; 74: 161-165.

[44] Tsiflikas I, Drosch T, Brodoefel H, et al. Diagnostic accuracy and image quality of cardiac dual-source computed tomography in patients with arrhythmia. *Int J Cardiol* 2010; 143: 79-85.

[45] Weustink AC, Meijboom WB, Mollet NR, et al. Reliable high-speed coronary computed tomography in symptomatic patients. *J Am Coll Cardiol* 2007; 50: 786-794.

[46] Weustink AC, Mollet NR, Neefjes LA, et al. Preserved diagnostic performance of dual-source CT coronary angiography with reduced radiation exposure and cancer risk. *Radiology* 2009; 252: 53-60.

[47] Xu Y, Tang L, Zhu X, et al. Comparison of dual-source CT coronary angiography and conventional coronary angiography for detecting coronary artery disease. *Int J Cardiovasc Imaging* 2010; 26: 75-81.

[48] Yang X, Gai L, Li P, et al. Diagnostic accuracy of dual-source CT angiography and coronary risk stratification. *Vasc Health Risk Manag* 2010; 6: 935-941.

[49] Zhang J, Liu T, Feng Y, et al. Diagnostic value of 64-slice dual-source CT coronary angiography in patients with atrial fibrillation: comparison with invasive coronary angiography. *Korean J Radiol* 2011; 12: 416-423.

[50] Sun Z, Jiang W. Diagnostic value of multislice CT angiography in coronary artery disease: A meta-analysis. *Eur J Radiol* 2006; 60: 279-286.

[51] Abdulla J, Abildstrom Z, Gotzsche O, et al. 64-multislice detector computed tomography coronary angiography as potential alternative to conventional coronary angiography: a systematic review and meta-analysis. *Eur Heart J* 2007; 28: 3042-3050.

[52] Mowatt G, Cook JA, Hillis GS, et al. 64-slicecomputed tomography angiography in the diagnosis and assessment of coronary artery disease: systematic review and meta-analysis. *Heart* 2008;94: 1386–1393.

[53] Vanhoenacker P, Heijenbrok-Kal M, Van Heste R, et al. Diagnostic performance of multidetector CT angiography for assessment of coronary artery disease: meta-analysis. *Radiology* 2007; 244: 419-428.

[54] Sun Z, Lin CH, Davidson R, et al. Diagnostic value of 64-slice CT angiography in coronary artery disease: A systematic review. *Eur J Radiol* 2008; 67: 78-84.

[55] Baumuller S, Leschka S, Desbiolles L, et al. Dual-source versus 64-section CT coronary angiography at lower heart rates: comparison of accuracy and radiation dose. *Radiology* 2009; 253: 56-64.

[56] Doninno R, Jacobs JE, Doshi JV, et al. Dual-source versus single-source cardiac CT angiography: comparison of diagnostic image quality. *AJR Am J Roentgenol* 2009; 192:1051-1056.

[57] Salavati A, Radmanesh F, Heidari K, et al. Dual-source computed tomography angiography for diagnosis and assessment of coronary artery disease: systematic review and meta-analysis. *J Cardiovasc Comput Tomogr* 2012; 6: 78-90.

[58] Budoff MJ, Dowe D, Jollis JG, et al. Diagnostic performance of 64-multidetector row coronary computed tomographic angiography for evaluation of coronary artery stenosis in individuals without known coronary artery disease: results from the prospective multicenter ACCURACY (Assessment by Coronary Computed Tomographic Angiography of Individuals Undergoing Invasive Coronary Angiography) trial. *J Am Coll Cardiol* 2008; 52:1724-1732.

[59] Miller JM, Rochitte CE, Dewey M, et al. Diagnostic performance of coronary angiography by 64-row CT. *N Engl J Med* 2008; 359:2324-2336.

[60] Hamon M, Biondi-Zoccai GG, Malagutti P, et al. Diagnostic performance of multislice spiral computed tomography of coronary arteries as compared with conventional

invasive coronary angiography: a meta-analysis. *J Am Coll Cardiol* 2006;48:1896-1910.

[61] Hausleiter J, Meyer T, Hadamitzky M, et al. Radiation dose estimates from cardiac multislice computed tomography in daily practice: impact of different scanning protocols on effective dose estimates. *Circulation* 2006;113:1305–1310.

[62] Primak AN, McCollough CH, Bruesewitz MR, Zhang J, Fletcher JG. Relationship between noise, dose, and pitch in cardiac multi-detector row CT. *Radiographics* 2006;26:1785–94.

[63] McCollough CH, Primak AN, Saba O, et al. Dose performance of a 64-channel dual-source CT scanner. *Radiology* 2007;243:775–84.

[64] Jakobs TF, Becker CR, Ohnesorge B, et al. Multislice helical CT of the heart with retrospective ECG gating: reduction of radiation exposure by ECG-controlled tube current modulation. *Eur Radiol* 2002; 12(5):1081–1086.

[65] Weustink AC, Neefjes LA, Kyrzopoulos S, et al. Impact of heart rate frequency and variability on radiation exposure, image quality, and diagnostic performance in dual-source spiral CT coronary angiography. *Radiology* 2009; 253: 672-680.

[66] Pflederer T, Rudofsky L, Ropers D, et al. Image quality in a low radiation exposure protocol for retrospectively ECG-gated coronary CT angiography. *AJR Am J Roentgenol* 2009; 192:1045-1050.

[67] Leschka S, Stolzmann P, Schmid F, et al. Low kilo voltage cardiac dual-source CT: attenuation, noise and radiation dose. *Eur Radiol* 2008; 18:1809-1817.

[68] Sun Z, Choo GH, Ng KH. Coronary CT angiography: current status and continuing challenges. *Br J Radiol* 2012; 85: 495-510.

[69] Sun Z, Ng KH. Prospective versus retrospective ECG-gated multislice CT coronary angiography: A systematic review of radiation dose and diagnostic accuracy. *Eur J Radiol* 2012; 81: e94-e100.

[70] von Ballmoos MW, Haring B, Juillert P, Alkadhi H. Meta-analysis: diagnostic performance of low-radiation-dose coronary computed tomography angiography. *Ann Intern Med* 2011; 154: 413-420.

[71] Sun Z, Ng KH. Diagnostic value of coronary CT angiography with prospective ECG-gating in the diagnosis of coronary artery disease: A systematic review and meta-analysis. *Int J Cardiovasc Imaging* 2012; 28: 2109-2119.

Chapter 6

320-Slice Coronary CT Angiography in Coronary Artery Disease: A Systematic Review of Diagnostic Value, Image Quality and Radiation Dose

Abstract

To perform a systematic review of the diagnostic value, image quality and radiation dose of 320-slice coronary CT angiography in the diagnosis of coronary artery disease when compared to invasive coronary angiography. A search of different databases was performed to identify studies investigating the diagnostic value of 320-slice coronary CT angiography in the diagnosis of coronary artery disease. Diagnostic value of 320-slice coronary CT angiography was compared to invasive coronary angiography and analysed at patient-, vessel- and segment-based assessment. Eleven studies met selection criteria and were included for analysis. The mean values and 95% confidence interval (CI) of sensitivity, specificity, positive predictive value and negative predictive value of 320-slice coronary CT angiography were 97% (95% CI: 93%, 100%), 90% (95% CI: 87%, 93%), 89% (95% CI: 85%, 94%) and 97% (95% CI: 93%, 100%), at patient-based analysis; 92% (95% CI: 86%, 98%), 95% (95% CI: 93%, 97%), 86% (95% CI: 79%, 92%) and 98% (95% CI: 96%, 99%), at vessel-based analysis; 90% (95% CI: 85%, 94%), 97% (95% CI: 95%, 99%), 85% (95% CI: 79%, 90%) and 98% (95% CI: 96%, 99%), at segment-based analysis, respectively. The mean effective dose of 320-slice coronary CT angiography was 10.5 mSv (95% CI: 6.8, 14.2 mSv). In patients with high heart rates, the mean radiation dose was 15.4 mSv (95% CI: 3.1, 27.6 mSv), which was significantly higher than the 5.2 mSv (95% CI: 2.6, 7.4 mSv) observed in patients with low heart rates. Diagnostic performance of 320-slice coronary CT angiography was independent of variable heart rates. In presence of high coronary calcium scores, specificity and positive predictive value was decreased when compared to the group with low calcium scores, although this did not reach significant difference. 320-slice coronary CT angiography has high diagnostic accuracy in the assessment of coronary artery disease, and its diagnostic performance remains high in the presence of high heart rates. High radiation dose associated with 320-slice coronary CT angiography is the main concern of this technology, and further dose-saving strategies should be implemented to minimize radiation exposure to patients.

Keywords: 320-slice CT, coronary CT angiography, diagnostic value, image quality, radiation dose

6.1. Introduction

Advances in multislice have made noninvasive imaging of the coronary artery disease (CAD) feasible with high diagnostic accuracy achieved. The main advantages of coronary CT angiography are its non-invasive nature, high specificity and negative predictive value compared with invasive coronary angiography, as reported in several previous studies using 64-slice and dual-source CT scanners [1-10]. Nonetheless, image quality of coronary CT angiography is still affected in patients with irregular heart rates, even with dual-source CT [8, 11].

Recently, a new generation of CT scanners has been introduced and it represents a significant advance from 64-slice technologies. The 320-slice CT is characterized by 320 slice detectors with a thickness of 0.5 mm and gantry rotation of 350 ms. It enables 16-cm coverage in the z-axis, thus, the whole heart can be covered in a single gantry rotation within one cardiac cycle [12]. Wide volume coronary CT angiography, in combination with prospective image acquisition allows for a significant decrease in scan time, resulting in decreased radiation dose and contrast medium when compared with retrospective helical gating protocols which require multiple heart beats. In addition, cardiac motion artefacts can be reduced and stair-step artefacts are eliminated with use of 320-slice CT.

Diagnostic performance of 320-slice coronary CT angiography has been investigated in previous studies based on low, irregular or high heart rates with satisfactory results achieved [13-16]. However, there is no systematic analysis of the diagnostic value of 320-slice coronary CT angiography with regard to the overall accuracy and effects of heart rates and calcium scores, as well as the associated radiation dose. The purpose of this chapter is to conduct a systematic review of the diagnostic value of 320-slice coronary CT angiography, according to the published studies in the literature.

6.2. Materials and Methods

6.2.1. Data Selection and Literature Searching

The literature search for relevant references was performed using different databases including Pubmed/Medline, ScienceDirect, Scopus and Embase to identify studies describing the diagnostic value of 320-slice coronary CT angiography in CAD between 2007 (320-slice CT was first introduced in 2007) and 2012 (last search was done in July 2012). The terms used for identification of references were '320-slice/320-detector row CT and coronary artery disease/stenosis', '320-slice coronary CT angiography', '320-slice CT angiography in CAD' and '320-slice CT in CAD'. The search was limited to include all the studies that have been published in the English language and were on human subjects. Case reports, conference abstracts, review articles, in vitro studies and articles investigating the coronary stents or bypass graft treatments were excluded from the analysis. In addition, the reference lists of identified articles were checked to obtain additional relevant articles.

Studies were included in the systematic review if they met all of the following criteria: (a) patients must be adults with suspected or known CAD who underwent 320-slice coronary CT angiography with use of retrospective ECG-gating or prospective ECG-triggering; (b) studies included at least 10 patients; (c) assessment or comparison of 320-slice CT coronary angiography with invasive coronary angiography was focused on the visualization of coronary arteries and detection or exclusion of CAD; (d) diagnostic value of 320-slice coronary CT angiography was clearly stated and addressed (lumen stenosis >50% as significant stenosis) when compared to invasive coronary angiography in terms of sensitivity, specificity, positive predictive value (PPV) and negative predictive value (NPV), either according to patients-based, or vessel-based or segments-based assessment.

6.2.2. Data Extraction

Data were extracted repeatedly based on study design and procedure techniques. The observer looked for the following characteristics in each study: year of publication; number of patients included in each study; mean age; mean heart rate (beats per minute-bpm); number of male patients; mean body mass index (BMI); number of patients receiving β–blockers; prevalence of suspected or known CAD; assessable coronary segments in each study; image quality assessment (qualitative or quantitative analysis); coronary artery calcium scores; radiation dose associated with 320-slice coronary CT angiography; diagnostic accuracy of 320-slice coronary CT angiography when compared to invasive coronary angiography in terms of the sensitivity, specificity, PPV, NPV and main factors affecting the visualization of coronary arteries or diagnostic performance. All diagnostic accuracy estimates referred to patient/vessel/segment-based assessment.

6.2.3. Image Quality Assessment

Quantitative and qualitative assessments of diagnostic image quality recorded in each study were analysed. Quantitative image quality was determined by measuring signal-to-noise ratio (SNR) and contrast-to-noise ratio (CNR) for comparisons among the studies. SNR was calculated as the mean Hounsfield unit (HU) of particular region of interest (ROI) divided by image noise. CNR was defined as the difference of attenuation values of the contrast enhancement at two different regions (eg. left ventricular chamber and left ventricular wall) and then divided by image noise. Image noise is a standard deviation, SD of HU measured at selected anatomical regions.

Qualitative assessment of image quality was carried out on a per-segment basis by using of three- to five-point Likert ranking scale. The coronary segments were analysed and the results were documented and categorized as percentage of assessable and non-assessable coronary segments. The classification of coronary segment was based on the descriptions of each score in Likert rank-scale. The coronary arteries were characterized into 15-17 segments according to the classification by American Heart Association (AHA) [17] and the extent of stenosis was evaluated in each segment with more than 50% coronary stenosis being defined as significant.

6.2.4. Statistical Analysis

All of the data were entered into SPSS (version 19.0) for analysis. Sensitivity, specificity, PPV and NPV estimates for each study were combined across studies using one sample test. Comparison was performed by Chi Square test using n-1 degree of freedom to test if there was any significant difference regarding the diagnostic value of 320-slice coronary CT angiography in CAD, between segment-based, vessel-based or patient-based assessment. Statistical hypotheses (2-tailed) were tested at the 5% level of significance.

6.3. Results

Figure 6.1 is the flow chart showing the review process to obtain these studies. After searching through these databases, we identified 120 articles, of which 22 potentially relevant articles were selected for full-text assessment. Eleven studies met our selection criteria, while the remaining 11 studies were excluded due to various reasons: contents duplicates (n=1); results focusing on the image quality and radiation dose, while information of diagnostic accuracy not presented (n=10).

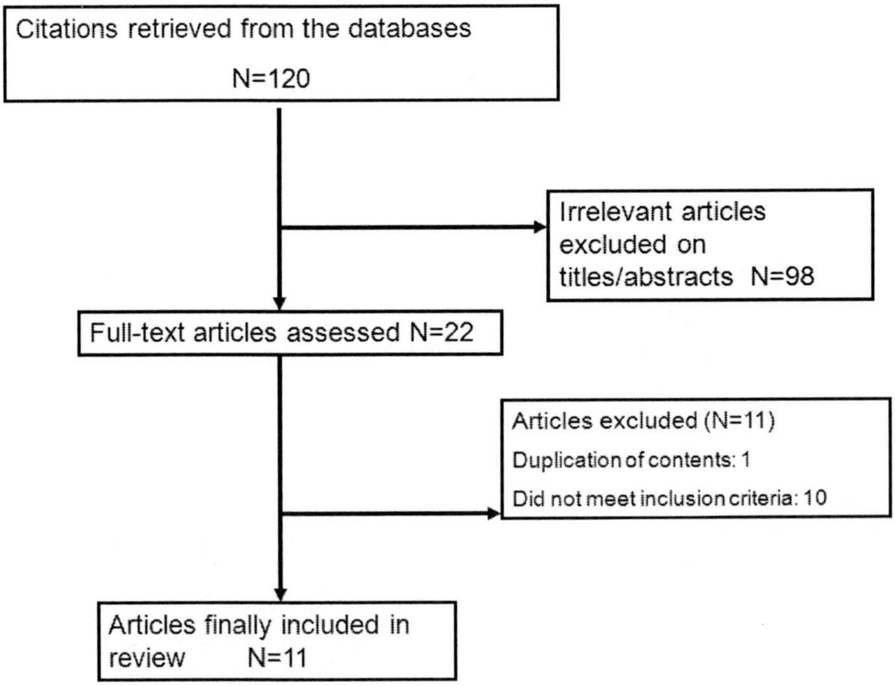

Figure 6.1. Flow chart shows the search strategy to obtain eligible references on 320-slice coronary CT angiography.

6.3.1. Study Characteristics

The characteristics of the eligible studies [14-16, 18-25] are presented in Table 6.1. The 11 studies enrolled 1258 patients (median, 64 patients, range, 37-240 patients). The mean age of the patients ranged from 45 to 68 years (median, 61 years). Of 11 studies, all were performed on 320-slice CT scanners (Toshiba Aquilion One, Toshiba Medical Systems, Japan) with temporal resolution of 175 ms. Coronary CT angiography was performed with prospective ECG-triggered scans in 9 studies, while in the remaining two studies, retrospectively ECG-gated scan was used [14, 25]. A combination of prospective triggering and retrospective gating (for left ventricular function assessment) scans was performed in one study [18]. A comparative analysis of the diagnostic performance of prospective triggering with retrospective gating was conducted in another study [19].

The percentage of assessable segments among these 11 studies with the mean value and 95% CI was 98% (95% CI: 97%, 99%). Coronary artery calcium scores were reported in 4 studies with the mean value being 350 (range, 180-653). The mean heart rate of patients during CT scan ranged from 56 to 88.4 bpm (median, 61.5 bpm). Beta-blocker was used in 4 studies, and no heart rate control was implemented in 2 studies, while in the remaining studies, detailed information about beta-blocker usage was not available.

6.3.2. Radiation Dose

Information about radiation dose was available in 10 studies, while in the remaining study, this was not reported [20]. The estimated mean effective dose and 95% CI was 10.5 mSv (95% CI: 6.8, 14.2 mSv), and it ranged from 3.1 to 23.2 mSv, depending on the scanning protocols used in each study (prospective triggering or retrospective gating). The mean effective dose for patients with high and low heart rates (more than 65 bpm versus less than 65 bpm) was 15.4 mSv (95% CI: 3.1, 27.6 mSv), 5.2 mSv (95% CI: 2.6, 7.4 mSv), respectively, indicating a significant difference ($p=0.05$) between these two groups.

Multiple heart beats reconstruction was performed in 4 studies, with effective dose reported in these studies [16, 19, 22, 25]. The effective dose of 320-slice coronary CT angiography was significantly higher in the multiple heartbeat groups (2- to 4-heart beat acquisition) than in the single heartbeat acquisition. In another study, the scanning field of view (FOV) was selected according to the patient's heart size [24]. The radiation dose in small-FOV (FOV=200 mm) scanning was found significantly higher than that in medium-FOV (FOV=320 mm) scanning, with no difference in image quality.

Prospective triggering was the most common approach used in these studies for dose reduction, while lower tube voltage such as 100 kVp was applied in 9 studies according to patients' BMI. Despite application of lower tube voltage among these studies, a direct comparison of effective dose between the 120 and 100 kVp groups was only performed in one study [22], with a dose reduction of 41% achieved in lower tube voltage group.

For the calculation of effective dose, different conversion coefficients were used in these studies, with a conversion coefficient of 0.014 and 0.017 mSv x mGy^{-1} x cm^{-1} applied in 4 and 2 studies, respectively. An updated conversion coefficient of 0.029 and 0.028 mSv x mGy^{-1} x cm^{-1} [26, 27] was used in 2 studies and 1 study, respectively [18, 20, 23]. In the remaining two studies, this information was not provided.

Table 6.1. Study characteristics of 320-slice coronary CT angiography in coronary artery disease

Studies	Year of publication	Detector collimation	No. Patients	No. of cases β blocker (%)	Mean age (yrs)	No. of Male	Heart Rate	Body mass index	Assessable segments (%)	Calcium score	Effective dose (mSv)
Dewey et al (14)	2009	320 x 0.5	30	56	61±10	21	59.9±6.6	26.2±4.7	100	384±742	4.2 (3.5 in low HR, 12.3 in high HR)
De Graaf et al (15)	2010	320 x 0.5	64	NA	61±16	34	60±11	26±2	99	184±223	10.8±2.8 (3.9±1.3 for HR<60, 6.0±3.0 for HR>60)
Xu et al (16)	2011	320 x 0.5	37	43	60±6	16	88.4±23.4	23.6±3	97	NA	13±4.7 (9±2.9 in 100 kV group, 15.2±4.1 in 120 kV group)
Gang et al (18)	2012	320 x 0.5	94	NA	65±10	65	74.2±11.2	23.9±3.5	93	NA	14.8±9.8 (7.1±7 for HR<70, 20.7±5.9 HR70-80, 23.7±5.4 HR>80)
Nasis et al (19)	2010	320 x 0.5	63	78	63.2±14	38	63±7	27.8±5	100	NA	10.6 (5.4 for PSG, 12.4 for RSG, 9.6 for single heartbeat, 14.2 for multiple heartbeat)
Qin et al (20) (retrospective gating)	2012	320 x 0.5	240	NA	45±16	156	56±6	21±7	99	NA	23.2±3.4
Qin et al (20) (Prospective gating)	2012	320 x 0.5	240	NA	45±20	163	56±8	22±9	99	NA	10±3.5
Uhera et al (21)	2012	320 x 0.5	106	0	64±12	72	65.2±15.2	NA	100	180	NA
Van Velzen et al (22)	2012	320 x 0.5	106	47	57±10	71	58±8	NA	96	NA	6.0±1.7 (12±4.5 for multiple heartbeat)
Gang et al (23)	2012	320 x 0.5	60	0	68±9	38	73.7±15.4	22.1±5.7	96	653 (413-1949)	12.5±9.4 (5.2±0.9 for HR<70, 22.6±5.2 for HR>70)

Studies	Year of publication	Detector collimation	No. Patients	No. of cases β blocker (%)	Mean age (yrs)	No. of Male	Heart Rate	Body mass index	Assessable segments (%)	Calcium score	Effective dose (mSv)
Zhang et al (24) (premature beat group)	2012	320 x 0.5	50	NA	61±10.7	NA	77.2±12.1	25.4±2.9	100	NA	14.6±1.4
Zhang et al (24) (control group)	2012	320 x 0.5	50	NA	57.8±10 .4	NA	58.7±4.7	25.5±2.6	100	NA	3.1±2.4
Pelliccia et al (25)	2012	320 x 0.5	118	NA	61±10	78	NA	25.1±6.6	100	NA	3.1±2.3/(2.1±1.1 for single heartbeat 4.2±2.9 for multiple heartbeat)

HR-heart rate, NA-not available, PSG-prospective ECG-gating, RSG-retrospective ECG-gating.

Table 6.2. Mean value of sensitivity, specificity, PPV and NPV of 320-slice coronary CT angiography according to patient-, vessel and segment-based assessment

Factors to be assessed		Sensitivity (95% CI)	Specificity (95% CI)	Positive predictive value (95% CI)	Negative predictive value (95% CI)
Patient-based analysis		97% (93%, 100%)	90% (87%, 93%)	89% (85%, 94%)	97% (93%, 100%)
Vessel-based analysis		92% (86%, 98%)	95% (93%, 97%)	86% (79%, 92%)	98% (96%, 99%)
Segment-based analysis		90% (85%, 94%)	97% (95%, 99%)	85% (79%, 90%)	98% (96%, 99%)
Heart rates	<65 bpm	88% (70%, 100%)	98% (98%, 98%)	83% (67%, 99%)	99% (97%, 100%)
	>65 bpm	86% (62%, 100%)	97% (95%, 99%)	82% (72%, 92%)	99% (97%, 100%)
Coronary calcium scores	Low CAC	79% (35%, 96%)	99% (99%, 99%)	84% (55%, 100%)	98% (95%, 100%)
	High CAC	90% (66%, 100%)	90% (70%, 100%)	79% (53%, 100%)	97% (93%, 100%)

bpm-beats per minute, CAC: coronary calcium score, CI-confidence interval, PPV-positive predictive value, NPV-negative predictive value.

6.3.3. Image Quality Assessment

A 15-, 16- and 17-segment AHA system was used in 5, 1 and 4 studies, respectively, while in the remaining study, this was not provided. Subjective assessment of 320-slice coronary CT angiography was performed in all studies with 2 observers blinded to the results of invasive coronary angiography assessing the image quality in 10 studies, while in the remaining study, only one observed assessed the coronary CT angiographic images. In contrast, invasive coronary angiographic images were evaluated by one observer in nearly half of the studies (45%), while two observers were involved in the assessment of angiographic images in 4 studies. Three observers were involved in the image analysis in one study, while in the remaining study, the information was not available. Quantitative assessment of image quality was not used in all of the studies, thus SNR or CNR was not available for analysis.

6.3.4. Diagnostic Value of 320-Slice Coronary CT Angiography

Of 11 studies, evaluation of 320-slice coronary CT angiography in CAD at patient-based assessment was available in 9 studies with 13 comparisons, as two studies involved comparative analysis of the diagnostic value of coronary CT angiography between patients with different heart rates. The mean values and 95% CI of the sensitivity, specificity, PPV and NPV of 320-slice coronary CT angiography were 97% (95% CI: 93%, 100%), 90% (95% CI: 87%, 93%), 89% (95% CI: 85%, 94%) and 97% (95% CI: 93%, 100%), respectively (Table 6.2). There was no significant difference in the diagnostic value of 320-slice CT coronary angiography between patients with high and low heart rates ($p>0.05$).

Evaluation of 320-slice coronary CT angiography in CAD at vessel-based assessment was available in 8 studies with 10 comparisons as one study involved comparison of the effect of heart rates on diagnostic value. The mean values and 95% CI of the sensitivity, specificity, PPV and NPV of 320-slice coronary CT angiography were 92% (95% CI: 86%, 98%), 95% (95% CI: 93%, 97%), 86% (95% CI: 79%, 92%) and 98% (95% CI: 96%, 99%), respectively (Table 6.2).

Evaluation of 320-slice coronary CT angiography in CAD at segment-based analysis was available in 11 studies with 25 comparisons, as 5 studies involved multiple comparisons. The mean values and 95% CI of the sensitivity, specificity, PPV and NPV of 320-slice coronary CT angiography were 90% (95% CI: 85%, 94%), 97% (95% CI: 95%, 99%), 85% (95% CI: 79%, 90%) and 98% (95% CI: 96%, 99%), respectively (Table 6.2).

6.3.5. Effect of Heart Rate on Diagnostic Value

Four studies investigated the effect of different heart rates on the diagnostic value of 320-slice coronary CT angiography, at segment-based analysis. Table 6.2 shows the mean values of sensitivity, specificity, PPV and NPV in patients with high and low heart rates. As shown in the table, there was no significant difference in the diagnostic performance between these two groups ($p>0.05$).

6.3.6. Effect of Coronary Artery Calcium on Diagnostic Value

Three studies provided coronary calcium scores and investigated their corresponding effects on diagnostic performance of 320-slice coronary CT angiography. Results showed that there was no significant difference in the diagnostic value between patients with low calcium scores and those with high calcium scores ($p>0.05$), although the specificity and PPV was decreased in the presence of high calcium score, as shown in Table 6.2.

Discussion

This systematic review has three findings which are considered important and valuable from a clinical perspective. Firstly, 320-slice coronary CT angiography has high diagnostic value in the detection of coronary stenosis, even in patients with high or irregular heart rates. In particular, high specificity (>90%) and very high negative predictive value (>97%) indicate that 320-slice coronary CT angiography can be used as a reliable modality to exclude significant coronary stenosis. Secondly, diagnostic performance of 320-slice coronary CT angiography is independent of heart rates, thus, patients with high or irregular hearts will benefit from this new technique. Thirdly, radiation dose associated with 320-slice coronary CT angiography is relatively high, and the dose value depends on the protocols used in performing coronary CT angiography scans.

The use of 320-slice CT makes it possible to image the whole heart in one heartbeat. This eliminates "stair-step" artefacts that are observed during 64-slice cardiac CT scans. Full cardiac coverage with one gantry rotation allows for evaluation of coronary arteries in patients with arrhythmias, such as with atrial fibrillation. In the presence of arrhythmias, an irregular R-R interval results in discontinuous imaging to the through plane with banding artefacts. Such images would impair the diagnostic accuracy of coronary CT angiography for assessment of the coronary lumen, leading to false diagnosis [28-30]. The imaging principle of 320-slice CT is different from previous generations of multislice CT scanners as there is no need to piece together image sub-volumes acquired over several heartbeats (normally 4-5 heartbeats for 64-slice coronary CT angiography) to reconstruct the entire cardiac volume. Furthermore, an arrhythmia rejection algorithm has been developed for 320-slice coronary CT angiography [13], thus, 320-slice CT can be used with increased reliability in imaging patients with irregular or high heart rates.

Although only 11 studies were analysed in this systematic review, patients with different heart rates or atrial fibrillation were included. High diagnostic value of sensitivity, specificity and negative predictive value (>90%) has been achieved at per-patient, vessel- and segment-based analysis. The results are compared favourably to the studies using 64-slice and dual-source coronary CT angiography [31-35]. The mean assessable segments of 98% by 320-slice coronary CT angiography also show that only a small percentage of coronary segments are non-diagnostic according to the 15- and 17-segment classification system. These findings suggest the improved diagnostic accuracy of 320-slice coronary CT angiography over 64-slice coronary CT angiography (both single-source and dual-source CT coronary angiography).

Prospective ECG-triggering with non-helical scan was used a long time ago with electron-beam CT for purpose of calcium scoring; however, it was recommended recently for cardiac CT imaging, and this imaging protocol is increasingly reported in the literature due to its resultant very low radiation dose. It has been widely reported that prospective ECG-triggering protocol reduces radiation dose significantly compared to the conventional retrospective ECG-gating protocol, with a dose reduction ranging from 76% to 83% [36-39]. The mean effective radiation dose for prospectively ECG-triggered coronary CT angiography in patients with a low and regular heart rate has been reported to range from 2.7 mSv to 4.5 mSv, according to several systematic reviews [40-42]. The mean effective dose of 320-slice coronary CT angiography in this analysis was 10.5 mSv, and this high dose value is due to inclusion of patients with high or irregular heart rates among these studies. When comparing the effective dose in patients with low heart rates to those with high heart rates, it was found that the mean effective dose was reduced to 5.2 mSv in the low heart rate group, which is similar to the range reported in the literature. Therefore, dose-saving strategies should be implemented in patients with high heart rates when undergoing 320-slice coronary CT angiography.

It is well-known that coronary arteries with severe calcification can lead to misdiagnosis of the extent of the plaques and degree of lumen stenosis due to blooming artefacts [43]. Calcified plaques were reported to be the most significant factor that affected diagnostic accuracy and coronary CT image quality, with more non-assessable segments observed in coronary artery with extensive calcification (Agatston calcium score >100) [44]. This analysis did not show significant difference in the diagnostic value of 320-slice coronary CT angiography between low and high coronary calcium scores. This is because the single gantry rotation of 320-slice CT reduced the blooming artefacts resulting from heavily calcified plaques. Despite high diagnostic value in patients with high calcium scores, the specificity and positive predictive value were decreased to some extent. Therefore, severe calcification still remains a factor compromising the diagnostic performance of 320-slice coronary CT angiography.

Some limitations exist in this analysis. Firstly, publication bias may have affected the results since we just included articles in English and excluded non-English references. Secondly, only a very small number of studies were eligible according to the selection criteria, as most of the currently available studies focused on the comparison of image quality and radiation dose without addressing the diagnostic accuracy of coronary CT angiography. Thirdly, among these eligible studies, not all of them provided detailed information regarding the diagnostic performance of coronary CT angiography. Thus, only a systematic review was performed, and meta-analysis of the studies could not be conducted.

In conclusion, this systematic review shows that 320-slice coronary CT angiography has high diagnostic accuracy in the diagnosis of coronary artery disease. There is no significant difference between patients with low and high heart rates in terms of the diagnostic performance, thus, 320-slice coronary CT angiography can be reliably used to diagnose patients with high or irregular heart rates. High radiation dose is associated with 320-slice coronary CT angiography; therefore, future studies with inclusion of dose-saving strategies should be conducted to minimize the radiation dose while achieving diagnostic images.

References

[1] Leber AW, Knez A, von Ziegler F, et al. Quantification of obstructive and nonobstructive coronary lesions by 64-slice computed tomography: A comparative study with quantitative coronary angiography and intravascular ultrasound. *J Am Coll Cardiol* 2005; 46: 147-54.

[2] Leschka S, Alkadhi H, Plass A, et al. Accuracy of MSCT coronary angiography with 64-slice technology: first experience. *Eur Heart J* 2005, 26: 1482-1487.

[3] Plass A, Grunenfelder J, Leschka S, et al. Coronary artery imaging with 64-slice computed tomography from cardiac surgical perspective. *Eur J Radiol* 2006; 30: 109-116.

[4] Raff GL, Gallagher MJ, O'Neill WW, et al. Diagnostic accuracy of non-invasive coronary angiography using 64-slice spiral computed tomography. *J Am Coll Cardiol* 2005, 46: 552-557.

[5] Flohr TG, McCollough CH, Bruder H, et al. First performance evaluation of a dual-source CT (DSCT) system. *Eur Radiol* 2006; 16(2):256–268.

[6] Plass A, Azemaj N, Scheffel H, et al. Accuracy of dual-source computed tomography coronary angiography: evaluation with a standardised protocol for cardiac surgeons. *Eur J Cardiothorac Surg* 2009; 36(6):1011–1017.

[7] Achenbach S, Ropers D, Kuettner A, et al. Randomized comparison of 64-slice single- and dual-source computed tomography coronary angiography for the detection of coronary artery disease. *JACC Cardiovasc Imaging* 2008; 1: 177-186.

[8] Brodoefel H, Burgstahler C, Tsiflikas I, et al. Dual-source CT: effect of heart rate, heart rate variability, and calcification on image quality and diagnostic accuracy. *Radiology* 2008; 247: 346-355.

[9] Chen H, Fang X, Hu X, et al. Efficacy of dual-source CT coronary angiography in evaluating coronary stenosis: initial experience. *Clin Imaging* 2010; 34: 165-171.

[10] Xu Y, Tang L, Zhu X, et al. Comparison of dual-source CT coronary angiography and conventional coronary angiography for detecting coronary artery disease. *Int J Cardiovasc Imaging* 2010; 26: 75-81.

[11] Bastarrika G, Arraiza M, Arias J, et al. Dual-source CT coronary angiography: image quality and optimal reconstruction interval. *Radiologia* 2009;51: 376–384.

[12] Rybicki F, Otero H, Steigner M, et al. Initial evaluation of coronary images from 320-detector row computed tomography. *Int J Cardiovasc Imaging* 2008; 24: 535-546.

[13] Pasricha SS, Nandurkar D, Seneviratne SK, et al. Image quality of coronary 320-MDCT in patients with atrial fibrillation: Initial experience. *AJR Am J Roentgenol* 2009; 193: 1514-1521.

[14] Dewey M, Zimmermann E, Deissenrieder F, et al. Noninvasive coronary angiography by 320-row computed tomography with lower radiation exposure and maintained diagnostic accuracy: comparison of results with cardiac catheterization in a head-to-head pilot investigation. *Circulation* 2009; 120: 867-875.

[15] de Graaf FR, Schuijf JD, van Velzen JE, et al. Diagnostic accuracy of 320-row multidetector computed tomography coronary angiography in the non-invasive evaluation of significant coronary artery disease. *Eur Heart J* 2010; 31: 1908-1915.

[16] Xu L, Yang L, Fan Z, et al. Diagnostic performance of 320-detector CT coronary angiography in patients with atrial fibrillation: preliminary results. *Eur Radiol* 2011; 21: 936-943.

[17] Austen WG, Edwards JE, Frye RL, et al. Report of the ad hoc committee for grading of coronary artery disease. A reporting system on patients evaluated for coronary artery disease. *Am Heart Assoc* 1975; 5-40.

[18] Sun G, Li M, Jiang XS, et al. 320-detector row CT coronary angiography: effects of heart rate and heart rate variability on image quality, diagnostic accuracy and radiation exposure. *Br J Radiol* 2012; 85: e388-394.

[19] Nasis A, Leung MC, Antonis PR, et al. Diagnostic accuracy of noninvasive coronary angiography with 320-detector row computed tomography. *Am J Cardiol* 2010; 106: 1429-1435.

[20] Qin J, Liu LY, Fang Y, et al. 320-detector CT coronary angiography with prospective and retrospective electrocardiogram gating in a single heartbeat: comparison of image quality and radiation dose. *Br J Radiol* 2012; 85: 945-951.

[21] Uehara M, Takaoka H, Kobayashi Y, Funabashi N. Diagnostic accuracy of 320-slice computed tomography for detection of significant coronary artery stenosis in patients with various heart rates and heart rhythms compared with conventional coronary angiography. *Int J Cardiol* (Epub ahead of print) doi:10.1016/j.ijcard.2012.02.017.

[22] van Velzen JE, de Graaf FR, Kroft LJ, et al. Performance and efficacy of 320-row computed tomography coronary angiography in patients presenting with acute chest pain: results from a clinical registry. *Int J Cardiovasc Imaging* 2012; 28: 865-876.

[23] Gang S, Min L, Li L, et al. Evaluation of CT coronary artery angiography with 320-row detector CT in a high-risk population. *Br J Radiol* 2012; 85: 562-570.

[24] Zhang T, Bai J, Wang W, Wang D, Shen B. Preliminary study of prospective ECG-gated 320-detector CT coronary angiography in patients with ventricular premature beats. *Plos One* 2012; 7: e38430.

[25] Pelliccia F, Pasceri V, Evangelista A, et al. Diagnostic accuracy of 320-row computed tomography as compared with invasive coronary angiography in unselected, consecutive patients with suspected coronary artery disease. *Int J Cardiovasc Imaging* (Epub ahead of print) DOI 10.1007/s10554-012-0095-4.

[26] Einstein AJ, Elliston CD, Arai AE, et al. Radiation dose from single-heart beat coronary CT angiography performed with a 320-detector row volume scanner. *Radiology* 2010;254:698–706.

[27] Gosling O, Loader R, Venables P, Rowles N, Morgan-Hughes G, Roobottom C. Cardiac CT: are we underestimating the dose? A radiation dose study utilising the2007 ICRP tissue weighting factors and a cardiac specific scan volume. *Clin Radiol* 2010;65:1013–17.

[28] Tsiflikas I, Drosch T, Brodoefel H, et al. Diagnostic accuracy and image quality of cardiac dual-source computed tomography in patients with arrhythmia. *Int J Cardiol* 2010;143:79–85.

[29] Cademartiri F, Mollet NR, Runza G, et al. Improving diagnostic accuracy of MDCT coronary angiography in patients with mild heart rhythm irregularities using ECG editing. *AJR Am J Roentgenol* 2006;186:634–8.

[30] Brodoefel H, Reimann A, Burgstahler C, et al. Noninvasive coronary angiography using 64-slice spiral computed tomography in an unselected patient collective: effect of

heart rate, heart rate variability and coronary calcifications on image quality and diagnostic accuracy. *Eur J Radiol* 2008;66:134–141.

[31] Sun Z, Lin CH, Davidson R, et al. Diagnostic value of 64-slice CT angiography in coronary artery disease: A systematic review. *Eur J Radiol* 2008; 67: 78-84.

[32] Abdulla J, Abildstrom Z, Gotzsche O, et al. 64-multislice detector computed tomography coronary angiography as potential alternative to conventional coronary angiography: a systematic review and meta-analysis. *Eur Heart J* 2007; 28: 3042-3050.

[33] Mowatt G, Cook JA, Hillis GS, et al. 64-slicecomputed tomography angiography in the diagnosis and assessment of coronary artery disease: systematic review and meta-analysis. *Heart* 2008;94: 1386–1393.

[34] Guo SL, Guo YM, Zhai YN, et al. Diagnostic accuracy of first generation dual-source computed tomography in the assessment of coronary artery disease: a meta-analysis from 24 studies. *Int J Cardiovasc Imaging* 2011; 27: 755-771.

[35] Salavati A, Radmanesh F, Heidari K, et al. Dual-source computed tomography angiography for diagnosis and assessment of coronary artery disease: systematic review and meta-analysis. *J Cardiovasc Comput Tomogr* 2012; 6: 78-90.

[36] Shuman WP, Branch KR, May JM, et al. Prospective versus retrospective ECG gating for 64-detector CT of the coronary arteries: comparison of image quality and patient radiation dose. *Radiology* 2008; 248(2):431–437.

[37] Huang B, Li J, Law MWM, Zhang J, Shen Y, Khong PL. Radiation dose and cancer risk in retrospectively and prospectively ECG-gated coronary angiography using 64-slice multidetector CT. *Br J Radiol* 2010; 83: 152-158.

[38] Stolzmann P, Goetti R, Baumueller S, et al. Prospective and retrospective ECG-gating for CT coronary angiography perform similarly accurate at low heart rates. *Eur J Radiol* 2011; 79: 85-91.

[39] Hong YJ, Kim SJ, Lee SM, et al. Low-dose coronary computed tomography angiography using prospective ECG-triggering compared to invasive coronary angiography. *Int J Cardiovasc Imaging* 2011; 27: 425-431.

[40] von Ballmoos MW, Haring B, Juillert P, Alkadhi H. Meta-analysis: diagnostic performance of low-radiation-dose coronary computed tomography angiography. *Ann Intern Med* 2011; 154: 413-420.

[41] Sun Z, Ng KH. Diagnostic value of coronary CT angiography with prospective ECG-gating in the diagnosis of coronary artery disease: A systematic review and meta-analysis. *Int J Cardiovasc Imaging*2012; 28: 2109-2119.

[42] Sun Z, Ng KH. Prospective versus retrospective ECG-gated multislice CT coronary angiography: A systematic review of radiation dose and diagnostic accuracy. *Eur J Radiol* 2012; 81: e94-e100.

[43] Budoff MJ, Dowe D, Jollis JG, et al. Diagnostic performance of 64-multidetector row coronary computed tomographic angiography for evaluation of coronary artery stenosis in individuals without known coronary artery disease: results from the prospective multicenter ACCURACY (Assessment by Coronary Computed Tomographic Angiography of Individuals Undergoing Invasive Coronary Angiography) trial. *J Am Coll Cardiol* 2008; 52:1724-1732.

[44] Rixe J, Rolf A, Conradi G, et al. Detection of relevant coronary artery disease using dual-source computed tomography in a high probability patient series: comparison with invasive angiography. *Circ J* 2009;73:316–22.

Chapter 7

Coronary CT Angiography in Coronary Artery Disease: A Systematic Review of Research Directions

Abstract

To investigate the research directions of coronary CT angiography in the diagnosis of coronary artery disease, based on a systematic review of the literature. A search of articles on coronary CT angiography in the diagnosis of coronary artery disease was performed during a seven-year-period between 2005 and 2011 from five main radiology journals namely, Radiology, American Journal of Roentgenology, European Radiology, European Journal of Radiology and British Journal of Radiology. Analysis of the references was focused on the research directions of coronary CT angiography with regard to the type of studies in terms of diagnostic value, application of dose-reduction strategies and resultant effective radiation doses with use of these techniques. One hundred and eighty seven studies were identified to meet the selection criteria and were included in the analysis. Prior to 2007, research was focused on the diagnostic value of coronary CT angiography, but since 2008 more attention has been given to the radiation dose reduction. Radiation dose was reported in 97 studies, representing 52% of total studies published in the five radiology journals. Various dose-saving strategies have been implemented, and prospective ECG-triggering and high pitch techniques were found to be the most effective approaches for radiation dose reduction, with resultant mean effective dose being 3.8 ± 1.8 mSv and 1.4 ± 0.6 mSv. This analysis shows that the current research in coronary CT angiography has shifted from the previous focus on diagnostic accuracy in coronary artery disease to the more emphasis on the radiation dose reduction. This change of research directions indicates the increased awareness of radiation dose associated with coronary CT angiography in the literature. The effective dose has been achieved through employing dose-reduction techniques with dose levels similar to, or lower than those from invasive coronary angiography.

Keywords: Coronary artery disease, coronary CT angiography, diagnostic value, multislice computed tomography, radiation dose

7.1. Introduction

Coronary artery disease (CAD) is the leading cause of morbidity and mortality in many advanced countries and its prevalence is increasing among developing countries [1, 2]. According to recent World Health Organization statistics for 2007, cardiovascular deaths account for 33.7% of all deaths worldwide, whereas cancer represents 29.5%, other chronic diseases 26.5%, injury 7%, and communicable diseases 4.6% [3].

CAD is the leading cause of cardiovascular death throughout the world. In light of the current global focus on healthcare utilization, costs, and quality, it is essential to monitor and understand the magnitude of healthcare delivery and costs, as well as the quality of healthcare delivery in relation to the CAD.

Invasive coronary angiography (ICA) is widely used as a reliable technique to diagnose CAD because of its superior spatial and temporal resolution. However, it is an invasive and expensive procedure with associated small percentage of morbidity and mortality [4]. As an alternative to ICA, coronary CT angiography has been increasingly used for the investigation of suspected CAD, and rapid technological developments of multislice CT (MSCT) have led to both improved spatial and temporal resolution [5-7].

Studies have shown that coronary CT angiography has a high diagnostic accuracy for the detection of significant CAD (≥50% lumen stenosis) when compared to ICA [8-11], and in selected patients, coronary CT angiography is recommended as a reliable alternative to ICA in the diagnosis of CAD.

Despite promising results having been achieved with coronary CT angiography, it has the disadvantage of high radiation dose, which leads to the concern of radiation-associated risks [12, 13]. It is generally agreed that CT is an imaging modality with high radiation exposure, as it contributes up to 70% radiation dose of all radiological examinations, although it comprises only 15% of all radiological examinations. Radiation-induced malignancy resulting from CT scan is a major issue that has raised serious concern in the medical field and this has been addressed by the National Research Council of the United States [14]. It is reported that radiation dose from a CT scan has been significantly underestimated by the radiologists and physicians [12, 15].

Despite the increased awareness of radiation risk, many clinicians and researchers have not realized the amount of radiation exposure associated with coronary CT angiography, or the possibility of tailoring the scanning protocols to reduce radiation exposure to patients. Thus, the purpose of this chapter was to investigate the current research directions of coronary CT angiography in CAD, based on a systematic review of the literature that was published in five main radiology journals during a 7-year period between 2005 and 2011.

7.2. Materials and Methods

7.2.1. Reference Searching

A search of articles on coronary CT angiography in cardiac imaging was performed during a seven-year-period between 2005 and 2011 from five main radiology journals, Radiology, American Journal of Roentgenology (AJR), European Radiology (ER), European

Journal of Radiology (EJR) and British Journal of Radiology (BJR). The reason we set up our searching started in 2005 is because 64-slice CT was introduced in 2004. The keywords used in searching the references in each journal website included: MSCT in CAD, diagnostic value of CT coronary/MSCT angiography in CAD, coronary CT angiography and CT coronary angiography, prospective ECG-gating/triggering in cardiac imaging, cardiac CT with radiation dose reduction.

In addition, searching for relevant articles was conducted by electronically checking the monthly issue of each journal's publications, and eligible full-text articles were obtained for data extraction and analysis. Prospective and retrospective studies were included if they met the following criteria: (a) studies conducted on human subjects or phantom with use of MSCT or coronary CT angiography in coronary artery disease; (b) either coronary calcium scoring, or diagnosis of CAD, or prognostic value of CAD, or myocardial perfusion imaging must be addressed in each study; (c) coronary CT angiography in terms of retrospective ECG-gating or prospective ECG-triggering must be clearly stated in each study; (d) any strategies to reduce radiation dose must be provided. Since it is possible that many studies would not meet the third and fourth criteria, thus, studies were still eligible for inclusion in the analysis as long as they met the first two criteria. Exclusion criteria were: studies on coronary stenting or coronary artery bypass surgery; review articles or case reports; a letter or comment to the editor.

7.2.2. Data Extraction and Analysis

All articles were reviewed and extracted on study design and procedure techniques. The retrieved articles were assessed according to the selection criteria. The following characteristics in each study were identified: year of publication; type of scanning unit used for coronary CT angiography; type of studies in terms of prospective or retrospective studies; researcher background, e.g. radiologists, cardiologists, physicians or other healthcare professionals (for example, medical imaging specialists); number of research centers where studies were performed. In addition, more focus was given to look for the research directions of coronary CT angiography with the aim of seeking for information about application of dose-saving strategies. This included the common approaches for dose reduction: adjustments of kVp and mAs (tube current modulation, either anatomy-based or ECG-controlled tube current modulation); high pitch value; prospective ECG-triggering versus retrospective gating, and reconstruction algorithms for dose reduction.

7.2.3. Statistical Analysis

All continuous variables were expressed as mean value ± SD. Statistical tests were performed using SPSS V 19.0 (SPSS, Inc., Chicago, ILL). Comparisons were performed using one sample T test. A p value less than 0.05 was considered statistically significant difference.

7.3. Results

7.3.1. General Information

One hundred and eighty seven studies were identified to meet the selection criteria and were included in the analysis. One hundred and seventy nine studies were conducted at a single center, while the remaining 8 studies were performed at multicenters. The majority of these studies were published in the ER with the highest number of total publications being 76 articles (41%), and the least number of studies was found in the BJR with only 13 studies being identified (7%). For the remaining three journals, Radiology, AJR and EJR, the corresponding studies were 33, 33 and 32, respectively.

Analysis of author background indicates that most of the studies were performed by radiologists, followed by cardiologists, and other healthcare professionals such as physicians and medical imaging specialists. Radiologists accounted for 55% of the authors who performed the studies, while cardiologists represented 35% of the researchers who were in collaboration with radiologists as a research team in all of the studies, except in two studies published in ER and one study in BJR, where cardiologists alone conducted the research.

Of 187 studies, 170 were performed on patients (91%), and the remaining 17 studies were conducted on anthropomorphic phantoms with the aim of investigating the effect of heart rate on diagnostic image quality, or radiation dose or high pitch value on image quality. Ninety studies (48%) were performed to study the diagnostic value (82 studies) and prognostic value (8 studies) of coronary CT angiography in CAD, while the remaining studies were mainly focused on the radiation dose reduction.

Coronary CT angiography was compared with integrated single photon emission computed tomography (SPECT)/CT and positron emission tomography (PET)/CT in two studies to demonstrate the potential myocardial perfusion value of coronary CT angiography. Coronary CT angiography was compared with cardiac magnetic resonance imaging (MRI) in 8 studies with half of them published in the journal of ER. Six out of these 8 studies investigated the diagnostic value of coronary CT angiography with regard to the accuracy of assessing myocardial perfusion compared to cardiac MRI, with four studies showing that coronary CT angiography could accurately assess the extension and patterns of myocardial perfusion with low radiation dose. In the remaining two studies, coronary CT angiography was found to have limited ability to demonstrate hemodynamic change or myocardial perfusion compared to cardiac MRI. One study showed that combining coronary CT angiography with cardiac MRI had high diagnostic value in the diagnosis of CAD compared to ICA. The remaining study compared left ventricular function assessment using five different software tools on dual-source coronary CT angiography in comparison with cardiac MRI, with interchangeable results of left ventricular function assessment reported.

7.3.2. Type of Multislice CT Scanners

Variable MSCT scanners were used in these studies, with 64- or more slice-scanners representing the majority (87%) of the studies. Figure 7.1 shows the distribution of different generations of MSCT scanners that were identified in the analysis. Despite rapid technological developments of MSCT scanners, such as the increased availability of 256- and 320-slice CT, single-source 64-slice and dual-source 64-slice CT still dominated 79% of the coronary CT angiography studies.

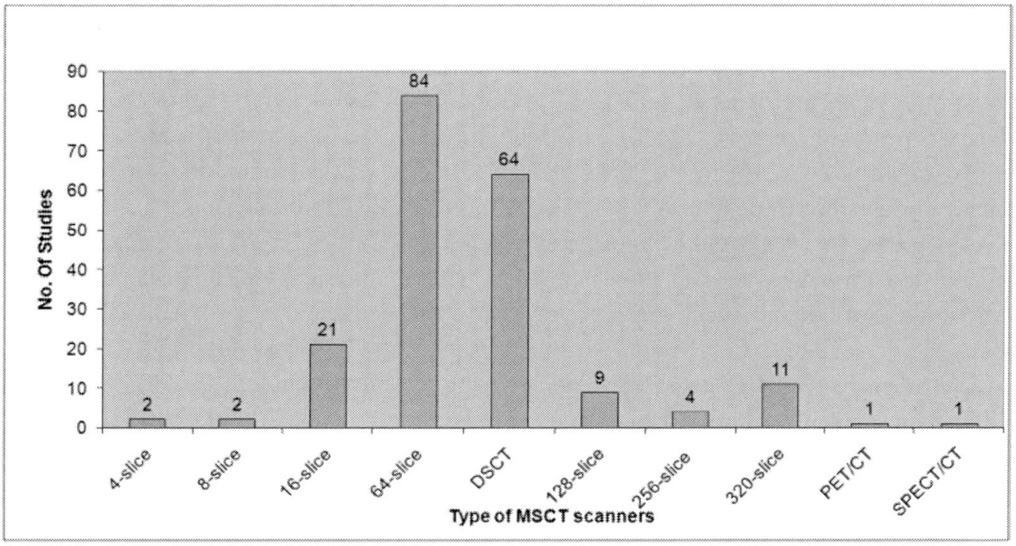

Figure 7.1. The number of studies performed with different generations of multislice CT scanners.

7.3.3. Research Directions of Coronary CT Angiography

Radiation dose issue has been addressed since 2007 in the publications of Radiology, AJR and BJR, while this has been addressed since 2008 in the publications of EJR. In comparison, radiation dose was first reported in 2 studies published in 2005 and 2006 in the journals of Radiology and ER, although more attention has been given to the dose issue since 2007. Prior to 2006 and 2007, the research was focused on the diagnostic value of coronary CT angiography in CAD, regardless of the studies performed with 8-slice, 16- or 64-slice CT scanners. From 2008, more and more studies started to address the reduction of radiation dose among these five radiology journals.

7.3.4. Dose-Saving Strategies

Various dose-saving strategies have been implemented in these studies, and these included adjustments of tube voltage (kVp), tube current (tube current modulation), high pitch value, prospective ECG-triggering versus retrospective ECG-gating, addition of padding in patients with high heart rate variability, and application of adaptive statistical iterative reconstruction algorithm for image noise reduction. Radiation dose was reported in 97 studies, representing 52% of total studies published in the five radiology journals. Of these 97 studies, 50% were published in the journal of ER.

Prospective ECG-triggering was the most commonly applied technique for dose reduction with 44 studies being reported among these five radiology journals. Of these 44 studies, a direct comparison between prospective ECG-triggering and retrospective gating was performed in 20 studies. The mean effective dose was 3.8 ± 1.8 mSv for prospective ECG-triggering, which is significantly lower (p<0.0001) than that acquired with retrospective ECG-gating, which is 15.1 ± 5.4 mSv.

ECG-controlled tube current modulation was the second most common approach that was utilized in 23 studies for dose reduction. However, the effective dose value was only reported in 17 studies, with the mean dose being 8.3 ± 2.4 mSv. Application of pitch (up to 3.4) in coronary CT angiography was reported in 10 studies with the mean effective dose being 1.4 ± 0.6 mSv. Lower kVp of 100 versus the standard 120 kVp was compared in 9 studies with the resultant mean effective dose of 4.7 ± 2.8 mSv for 100 kVp protocols, and 9.8 ± 5.3 mSv for 120 kVp protocols, leading to a dose reduction by 52%. Of these 9 studies, one study compared the 80 kVp with 100 kVp in patient with body mass index (BMI) less than 25 kg/m^2 with use of both prospective triggering and retrospective gating protocols. This resulted in much lower dose of 0.76 mSv with use of prospectively ECG-triggered and 4.3 mSv with use of retrospectively ECG-gated coronary CT angiography, although the 80 kVp protocol has higher image noise than the 100 kVp protocol. Figure 7.2 shows the mean effective dose associated with the above-mentioned commonly used strategies for dose reduction. As shown in the figure, prospective ECG-triggering and high pitch lead to the lowest doses when compared to other dose-saving strategies.

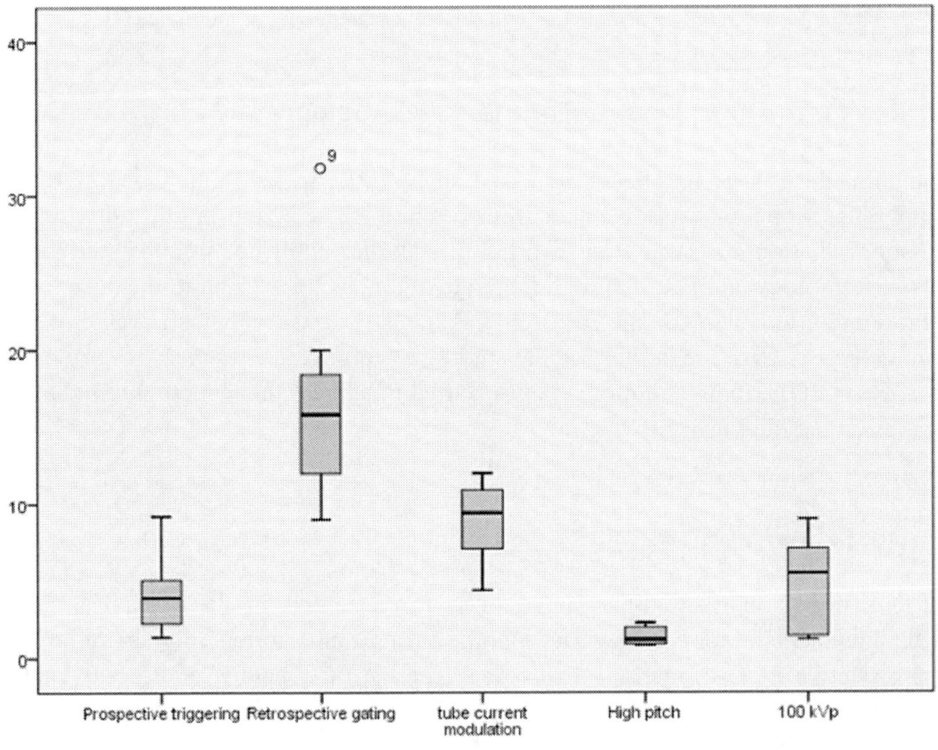

Figure 7.2. Box plot shows the mean effective dose associated with different dose-reduction techniques. Coronary CT angiography with use of high pitch and prospective ECG-triggering protocols lead to the lowest radiation dose.

Adaptive statistical iterative reconstruction (ASIR) was reported in three studies and the mean effective dose was less than 3.0 mSv, which is significantly lower than the traditional filtered back projection approach. A comparison of radiation dose with use of the International Commission on Radiological Protection (ICRP) 103 and ICRP 60 documents was conducted in two studies with a significant difference observed, indicating that the radiation dose was underestimated if dose calculation is based on the weighting factors that were reported in the ICRP 60.

Radiation dose corresponding to different heart rates was reported in four studies and the analysis shows that dual-source CT (DSCT) is superior to single-source CT in the diagnosis of CAD in patients with higher heart rates, with resultant lower doses. Padding was applied in one study performed with prospective ECG-triggering. The purpose of adding padding is to provide additional phase information to compensate for variations in heart rate by adding time before and after the centre phase of the acquisition. Padding is described in the range of 0-200 ms and is added to both sides of the centre of the acquisition with padding 0 corresponding to a window of 100 ms scanning time and padding 100 corresponding to a window of 200 ms scanning time. In that study, the effective dose was 2.3 mSv for 0 padding, and dose increased to 3.8 mSv for 1-99 padding and 5.5 mSv for 100-150 padding.

The remaining study involved the investigation of the effect of adjusting the scan length of coronary CT angiography using the calcium scoring images instead of the scout view with regard to radiation dose. The effective dose associated with the calcium scoring-derived length (9.0 ± 0.6 mSv) was significantly lower than that using the scout view-derived length (10.7 ±1.2 mSv), corresponding to a radiation dose reduction of 16%.

Effective dose of coronary CT angiography was estimated by multiplying the dose length product (DLP) by a chest-specific with conversion coefficient of κ=0.014 or 0.017 mSv × mGy × cm^{-1} among these studies.

Discussion

This analysis presents three findings which are considered important for clinical application of coronary CT angiography in CAD. Firstly, there is a changing in research direction with a shift of focus from the previous diagnostic value of coronary CT angiography in CAD to an emphasis on radiation dose reduction. This indicates the increased awareness of radiation dose to patients during coronary CT angiography examinations. Secondly, more dose-saving strategies have been implemented to reduce radiation dose associated with coronary CT angiography while still maintaining diagnostic image quality. Of these strategies, prospective ECG-triggering and high pitch protocols represent the most effective approaches with a significant reduction of radiation dose compared to conventional retrospective gating or other approaches. Thirdly, coronary CT angiography performed with 64-slice CT (single-source or DSCT) dominated the majority of studies that were reviewed, and this indicates that 64-slice CT still plays a key role in the clinical diagnosis of CAD, despite the emergence of 256- or 320-slice CT.

Over the last decade a great deal of interest has been focused on the imaging and diagnosis of CAD using coronary CT angiography, due to its less invasive nature and improved spatial and temporal resolution. Moderate to high diagnostic accuracy was achieved with 64- or more slice CT, owing to further technical improvements [16-20]. These studies have indicated that coronary CT angiography has high accuracy for the diagnosis of CAD and could be used as an effective alternative to ICA in selected patients. However, coronary CT angiography has the disadvantage of high radiation dose which raises concerns for both clinicians and manufacturers. This is reflected in the changing research directions from the early research focus on the diagnostic value of coronary CT angiography in CAD to the increasingly reported studies on dose reduction, as demonstrated in this analysis.

Radiation dose is becoming a major issue for coronary CT angiography, since 64- or more-slice CT shows improved and promising results in the diagnosis of CAD [21-24]. It is estimated that in daily practice, effective dose of coronary CT angiography may reach up to 40 mSv in female patients if no dose-saving strategies are applied, and this is associated with radiation exposure to breast tissues [25]. The radiation risks associated with coronary CT angiography have raised serious concerns and have become a hot topic of debate in the literature in recent years [12, 13, 26]. The general view about radiation dose is that CT is associated with a risk of cancer development. The recent Biological Effects of Ionizing Radiation (BEIR) VII provides a framework for estimating cancer risk associated with radiation exposure from ionizing radiation [14]. According to the report, it is estimated that 1 in 2000 people will develop cancer due to an exposure of 10 mSv. Brenner and Hall [12] estimated that approximately 1.5% to 2% of all cancers in the United States may be caused by radiation exposure from CT examinations. Davies *et al* estimated that in the UK radiation from CT scans causes 800 cancers a year in women and 1300 in men [27]. Radiation exposure is especially important for young and female patients as radiation effects in young patients and women are more severe than in older individuals and in men, so that protection from overly high radiation doses are most important in young individuals. A recent study reported that one in 270 women aged 40 years who undergo coronary CT angiography will develop cancer [28]. Therefore, coronary CT angiography should be performed with dose-saving strategies whenever possible to reduce the radiation dose to patients.

One of the most effective approaches for dose reduction is adjustment of the tube current according to ECG signal, which is defined as ECG-controlled tube current modulation. This approach represents the most significant improvement in minimizing radiation exposure from coronary CT angiography. It has been reported that radiation dose can be reduced by 30%-50% through modulation of the tube current output to decrease the dose given during the systolic phase [29,30]. The estimated radiation dose reduction is similar to or less than that of an ICA examination with use of this dose saving strategy [29, 31]. The mean effective dose of ECG-controlled tube current modulation in this analysis is 8.3 mSv, and this is comparable to that of ICA, which is between 3-9 mSv [32].

Prospective ECG-triggered scans use the same technique as that used in electron-beam CT which is defined as the step-and-shoot method. The technique is initially used for quantitative assessment of coronary calcium burden, but recently it has been increasingly used for coronary CT angiography examinations. Unlike retrospective ECG-gating, prospective ECG-triggering allows for acquisition of data by selectively turning on the X-ray tube on only in the selected phase, triggered by the ECG signal, and turning it off during the rest of R-R cycle. In prospective ECG-triggering, exposure only occurs at the pre-defined cardiac phase instead of the continuous exposure during the entire cardiac cycle, thus leading to a significant reduction of radiation dose. Prospective ECG-triggering has been confirmed to be one of the most efficient techniques for radiation dose reduction in coronary CT angiography [33]. Use of prospective ECG-triggering with 64-slice or dual-source CT has been reported to reduce the effective radiation dose by up to 90% when compared to retrospective ECG-gating technique, with diagnostic image quality being achieved in more than 90% of the cases [34-40]. This is confirmed in this analysis as the mean effective dose of prospective triggering is 3.8 mSv, which is equivalent to or even lower than that of invasive coronary angiography.

Another effective method currently undertaken in coronary CT angiography to reduce radiation dose is to lower the tube voltage, since radiation dose varies with the square of the kVp. Modern CT scanners include tube voltages of 120 or 140 kVp, reflecting the settings most often resulting in adequate image quality. However, acquisition of cardiac CT images with 100 kVp, or even lower, is possible and has been suggested as an effective means to reduce radiation dose in coronary CT angiography [41, 42]. Up to 70% dose reduction has been reported in the literature when the X-ray tube voltage is decreased from 120 kVp to 100 kVp or even lower to 80 kVp [43-45]. This analysis shows that 52% dose reduction was observed in coronary CT angiography with use of 100 kVp when compared to the routine 120 kVp protocol, and this is consistent with the results reported in the literature. However, attention should be paid to changing the tube voltage as it is directly correlated with patient's BMI. Lowering tube voltage from 120 kVp to 100 or 80 kVp can be used when the patient's BMI is less than 25 kg/m^2. Therefore, tube voltage can be adjusted in cardiac CT angiography without affecting diagnostic image quality, and this should be applied whenever possible in clinical practice [46].

For coronary CT angiography, very low pitch values (0.2-0.4) are typically required for coronary data acquisition to ensure continuous z-axis coverage between image stacks reconstructed from consecutive cardiac cycles. The main disadvantage of this approach is higher radiation exposure since the table is advanced by less than one detector width during each gantry rotation, thus, same anatomic area is exposed to X-ray radiation during consecutive rotations of the gantry. Increasing pitch to a higher value was made possible with the development of the second generation of dual-source CT scanners, Siemens Definition Flash, which enabled acquisition of 128 slices simultaneously (flying focal spot) [47-50]. This DSCT mode allows coronary CT angiography to be performed at high pitch value of up to 3.4 with significant reduction of radiation dose. A high pitch was applied in 10 studies in this analysis with a mean effective dose of 1.4 mSv, and radiation dose less than 1.0 mSv was also reported in three studies, indicating the effectiveness of this dose-reduction approach. The new scan mode, with a superior temporal resolution of 75 ms, is regarded as an attractive alternative to invasive coronary angiography due to the very low dose and high image quality, although more studies based on a large cohort are required.

More recently, different iterative image reconstruction methods for reducing radiation dose without compromising image quality have been developed by all major CT manufacturers, and the method of ASIR represents a good example of dose reduction approach which was developed by the GE Healthcare [51, 52]. ASIR is an alternative to filtered back projection for image reconstruction in coronary CT angiography. ASIR incorporates statistical modelling to reduce image noise, which may allow preservation of image quality with reduced tube current, thereby resulting in lower radiation dose. Recent studies have shown that use of ASIR leads to up to 44% dose reduction compared to standard filtered back projection while maintaining diagnostic images [53, 54]. An effective dose less than 3.0 mSv was reported in three studies according to this analysis, and this demonstrates that ASIR represents a novel method of radiation dose reduction that appears additive to existing techniques.

The calculation of the effective dose of coronary CT angiography takes into account the biological effect of the radiation on the heart because each organ is given a tissue weighting depending on its individual susceptibility to the effects of ionizing radiation. The tissue weightings are derived from the ICRP documentation which focuses on all aspects of protection from ionizing radiation. In 2007, ICRP released the 103 publication updating the 16-year old ICRP 60 dataset, following the latest available scientific information of the biology and physics of radiation exposure, particularly the tissue weighting for breast tissue has increased from 0.05 to 0.12 [55]. The conversion factor used to calculate effective dose from coronary CT angiography has been upgraded from 0.014 to 0.028, thus, doses from coronary CT angiography could be significantly underestimated due to failure of using a cardiac specific conversion factor in the recent ICRP documentation [56, 57]. This is also confirmed in this analysis as the effective dose of coronary CT angiography calculated with ICRP 103 is 24% to 42% higher than that calculated with ICRP 60. Appropriate conversion factors are needed to reflect the current tissue weighting and accurately estimate effective dose.

Effective dose based on a conversion factor of 0.014 or 0.017 is only an estimate. The calculation of the effective dose in these studies is based on a method proposed by the European Working Group for Guidelines on Quality Criteria in CT [58], deriving radiation dose estimates from the product of the DLP and an organ weighting factor for the chest as the investigated anatomic region (k = 0.014 or 0.107 $mSv*mGy^{-1}*cm^{-1}$ averaged between male and female models from Monte Carlo simulations [59]. The DLP represents most closely the radiation dose received by an individual patient and may be used to set reference values for a given type of CT examination to help ensure patient doses at CT are as low as reasonably achievable. It is recommended that DLP should be recorded for each study and serve as the cornerstone of quality assurance efforts [60].

Some limitations exist in this review. Firstly, our searching for references only focused on the five main radiology journals. However, research articles on cardiac CT imaging are also published in cardiac journals such as European Heart Journal, Journal of American College of Cardiology, Circulation, American Journal of Cardiology and International Journal of Cardiovascular Imaging. Therefore, it is possible that some relevant references are not included in this analysis. Secondly, although tube current modulation is one of the most effective methods for radiation dose reduction, a number of studies did not report the actual effective dose, despite application of this technique in their studies. This emphasises the importance of awareness of radiation exposure to patients by physicians; thus, radiation dose values (volumetric CT dose index or dose length product) should be recorded in each study to enable comparison of dose-saving techniques between different studies. Thirdly, we tried to include as many references as possible that were available over the last seven years; however, some articles which were accepted for publication are excluded from the analysis. Finally, although this analysis shows that 64-slice coronary CT angiography dominated the majority of the studies, there is no doubt that more and more studies are being performed with latest models such as 256- and 320-slice CT scanners. Further research to include these studies is necessary.

In conclusion, this chapter based on a systematic review of the literature in five main radiology journals shows that the current research in coronary CT angiography has shifted from the previous focus on diagnostic accuracy in coronary artery disease to the more emphasis on the radiation dose reduction. This review also indicates that the increased awareness of radiation dose associated with coronary CT angiography in the literature. Various dose-saving strategies have been undertaken in the past few years to lower the radiation exposure to patients undergoing coronary CT angiography. Effective dose reduction has been achieved by employing techniques with radiation dose of around 10 mSv to as low as 1 mSv in some studies. It is important to note that the current effective doses from coronary CT angiography are at the level or even lower than those acquired from ICA. Therefore, according to this analysis, the achievements in radiation dose reduction in coronary CT angiography have been tremendous.

References

[1] Lloyd-Jones D, Adams RJ, Brown TM, et al. American Heart Association Statistics Committee and Stroke Statistics Subcommittee. Executive summary: heart disease and stoke statistics 2010 update: A report from the American Heart Association. *Circulation* 2010; 121: 948-954.

[2] Gaziano TA, Bitton A, Anand S, et al. Growing epidemic of coronary heart disease in low-and middle-income countries. *Curr Probl Cardiol* 2010; 35: 72-115.

[3] WHO. The World Health Report 2002: Reducing Risks, Promoting Healthy Life. Geneva: World Health Organization, 2002.

[4] Noto TJ Jr, Johnson LW, Krone R, et al. Cardiac catheterization 1990: a report of the registry of the Society for Cardiac Angiography and Interventions. (SCA&I). *Cathet Cardiovasc Diagn* 1991; 24:75–83.

[5] Nieman K, Oudkerk M, Rensing BJ, et al. Coronary angiography with multi-slice computed tomography. *Lancet* 2001; 357: 599-603.

[6] Kuettner A, Trabold T, Schroeder S, et al. Noninvasive detection of coronary artery lesions using 16-detector row multislice spiral computed tomography technology: initial clinical results. *J Am Coll Cardiol* 2004; 44: 1230-7.

[7] Pugliese F, Mollet NR, Runza G, et al. Diagnostic accuracy of non-invasive 64-slice CT coronary angiography in patients with stable angina pectoris. *Eur Radiol* 2006;16:575-582.

[8] Sun Z, Jiang W. Diagnostic value of multislice CT angiography in coronary artery disease: A meta-analysis. *Eur J Radiol* 2006; 60: 279-286.

[9] Miller JM, Rochitte CE, Dewey M, et al. Diagnostic performance of coronary angiography by 64-row CT. *N Engl J Med* 2008; 359: 2324-2336.

[10] Budoff MJ, Dowe D, Jollis JG, et al. Diagnostic performance of 64-multidetector row coronary computed tomographic angiography for evaluation of coronary artery stenosis in individuals without known coronary artery disease: results from the prospective multicenter ACCURACY (Assessment by Coronary Computed Tomographic Angiography of Individuals Undergoing Invasive Coronary Angiography) trial. *J Am Coll Cardiol* 2008;52:1724-1732.

[11] Meijboom WB, Meijs MFL, Schuijf JD, et al. Diagnostic accuracy of 64-slice computed tomography coronary angiography: a prospective multicenter, multivendor study. *J Am Coll Cardiol* 2008; 52:2135-2144.

[12] Brenner DJ, Hall EJ. Computed tomography—an increasing source of radiation exposure. *N Engl J Med* 2007; 357(22):2277–2284.

[13] Hausleiter J, Meyer T, Hermann F, et al. Estimated radiation dose associated with cardiac CT angiography. *JAMA* 2009; 301: 500-507

[14] Committee to Assess Health Risks from Exposure to Low Levels of Ionizing Radiation; Nuclear and Radiation Studies Board, Division on Earth and Life Studies, National Research Council of the National Academies. Health Risks From Exposure to Low Levels of Ionizing Radiation: BEIR VII Phase 2. Washington, DC: *The National Academies Press;* 2006.

[15] Lee CI, Haims AH, Monico EP, Brink JA, Forman HP. Diagnostic CT scans: assessment of patient, physician, and radiologist awareness of radiation dose and possible risks. *Radiology* 2004; 231(2):393–398.

[16] Sun Z, Lin CH, Davidson R, Dong C, Liao Y. Diagnostic value of 64-slice CT angiography in coronary artery disease: A systematic review. *Eur J Radiol* 2008; 67: 78-84.

[17] Vanhoenacker P, Heijenbrok-Kal M, Van Heste R, et al. Diagnostic performance of multidetector CT angiography for assessment of coronary artery disease: meta-analysis. *Radiology* 2007; 244: 419-428

[18] Abdulla J, Abildstrom Z, Gotzsche O, et al. 64-multislice detector computed tomography coronary angiography as potential alternative to conventional coronary angiography: a systematic review and meta-analysis. *Eur Heart J* 2007; 28: 3042-3050.

[19] Mowatt G, Cook JA, Hillis GS, et al. 64-slice computed tomography angiography in the diagnosis and assessment of coronary artery disease: systematic review and meta-analysis. *Heart* 2008;94: 1386–1393.

[20] Stein PD, Yaekoub AY, Matta F, Sostman HD. 64-slice CT for diagnosis of coronary artery disease: a systematic review. *Am J Med* 2008; 121: 715-725.

[21] Raff GL, Gallagher MJ, O'Neill WW, Goldstein JA. Diagnostic accuracy of non-invasive coronary angiography using 64-slice spiral computed tomography. *J Am Coll Cardiol* 2005, 46:552-557.

[22] Chao SP, Law WY, Kuo CJ, et al. The diagnostic accuracy of 256-row computed tomographic angiography compared with invasive coronary angiography in patients with suspected coronary artery disease. *Eur Heart J* 2010; 31: 1916-1923.

[23] Rybicki F, Otero H, Steigner M, et al. Initial evaluation of coronary images from 320-detector row computed tomography. *Int J Cardiovasc Imaging* 2008; 24:535-546.

[24] Dewey M, Zimmermann E, Deissenrieder ZF, et al. Noninvasive coronary angiography by 320-row computed tomography with lower radiation exposure and maintained diagnostic accuracy: comparison of results with cardiac catheterization in a head-to-head pilot investigation. *Circulation* 2009;120:867-875.

[25] Paul JF, Abada HT. Strategies for reduction of radiation dose in cardiac multislice CT. *Eur Radiol* 2007; 17:2028-2037.

[26] Raff GL, Chinnaiyan KM, Share DA, et al. Advanced Cardiovascular Imaging Consortium Co-Investigators. Radiation dose from cardiac computed tomography

before and after implementation of radiation dose-reduction techniques. *JAMA* 2009; 301:2340-2348.

[27] Davies HE, Wathen CG, Gleeson FV. Risks of exposure to radiological imaging and how to minimise them. *BMJ* 2011; 342: 589-593.

[28] Smith-Bindman R, Lipson J, Marcus R, et al. Radiation dose associated with common computed tomography examinations and the associated lifetime attributable risk of cancer. *Arch Intern Med* 2009; 169: 2078-2086.

[29] Jakobs TF, Becker CR, Ohnesorge B, et al. Multislice helical CT of the heart with retrospective ECG gating: reduction of radiation exposure by ECG-controlled tube current modulation. *Eur Radiol* 2002; 12: 1081-1086.

[30] Deetjen A, Mollmann S, Conradi G, et al. Use of automatic exposure control in multislice computed tomography of the coronaries: comparison of 16-slice and 64-slice scanner data with conventional coronary angiography. *Heart* 2007; 93: 1040-1043.

[31] Abada HT, Larchez C, Daoud B, Sigal-Cinqualbre A, Paul JF. MDCT of the coronary arteries: feasibility of low-dose CT with ECG-pulsed tube current modulation to reduce radiation dose. *AJR Am J Roentgenol* 2006; 186: S387-S390.

[32] Report of the United Nations Scientific Committee on the Effects of Atomic Radiation. *General Assembly Official Records.* 63rd Session. Suppl 46. 2008. www.undemocracy.com/A-63-398.pdf.

[33] Hsieh J, Londt J, Vass M, et al. Step-and-shoot data acquisition and reconstruction for cardiac X-ray computed tomography. *Med Phys* 2006; 33:4236-4248.

[34] Schoenhagen P. Back to the future: coronary CT angiography using prospective ECG triggering. *Eur Heart J* 2008; 29(2):153–154.

[35] Shuman WP, Branch KR, May JM, et al. Prospective versus retrospective ECG gating for 64-detector CT of the coronary arteries: comparison of image quality and patient radiation dose. *Radiology* 2008; 248: 431-437

[36] Hirai N, Horiguchi J, Fujioka C, et al. Prospective versus retrospective ECG-gated 64-detector coronary CT angiography: assessment of image quality, stenosis, and radiation dose. *Radiology* 2008; 248: 424-430.

[37] Earls J, Berman E, Urban B, et al. Prospectively gated transverse coronary CT angiography versus retrospectively gated helical CT technique: improved image quality and reduced radiation dose. *Radiology* 2008; 246: 742-753.

[38] Pontone G, Andreini D, Bartorelli AL, et al. Diagnostic accuracy of coronary computed tomography angiography: A comparison between prospective and retrospective electrocardiogram triggering. *J Am Coll Cardiol* 2009; 54: 346-355.

[39] Klass O, Jeltsch M, Feuerlein S, et al. Prospectively gated axial CT coronary angiography: preliminary experiences with a novel low-dose technique. *Eur Radiol* 2009; 19: 829-836.

[40] Sun Z, Ng KH. Prospective versus retrospective ECG-gated multislice CT coronary angiography: A systematic review of radiation dose and diagnostic accuracy. *Eur J Radiol* 2012; 81: e94-e100.

[41] Sun Z. Multislice CT angiography in cardiac imaging: prospective ECG-gating or retrospective ECG-gating? *Biomed Imaging Intervent J* 2010; 6(1) e4.

[42] Bae KT, Seeck BA, Hildebolt CF, et al. Contrast enhancement in cardiovascular MDCT: effect of body weight, height, body surface area, body mass index, and obesity. *AJR Am J Roentgenol* 2008;190:777–784.

[43] Feuchtner GM, Jodocy D, Klauser A, et al. Radiation dose reduction by using 100-kV tube voltage in cardiac 64-slice computed tomography: A comparative study. *Eur J Radiol* 2010; 75: e51-e56.

[44] Pflederer T, Rudofsky L, Ropers D, et al. Image quality in a low radiation exposure protocol for retrospectively ECG-gated coronary CT angiography. *AJR Am J Roentgenol* 2009; 192:1045-1050.

[45] Leschka S, Stolzmann P, Schmid F, et al. Low kilovoltage cardiac dual-source CT: attenuation, noise and radiation dose. *Eur Radiol* 2008; 18:1809-1817.

[46] Alkadhi H, Stolzmann P, Scheffel H, et al. Radiation dose of cardiac dual-source CT: the effect of tailoring the protocol of patient-specific parameters. *Eur J Radiol* 2008; 68: 385-391.

[47] Sun Z. Multislice CT angiography in coronary artery disease: technical developments, radiation dose and diagnostic value. *World J Cardiol* 2010; 26: 333-343.

[48] Achenbach S, Marwan M, Ropers D, et al. Coronary computed tomography angiography with a consistent dose below 1 mSv using prospectively electrocardiogram-triggered high-pitch spiral acquisition. *Eur Heart J* 2010; 31:340-346.

[49] Lell M, Marvan M, Schepis T, et al. Prospectively ECG-triggered high-pitch spiral acquisition for coronary CT angiography using dual source CT: technique and initial experience. *Eur Radiol* 2009; 19:2576-2583.

[50] Ertel D, Lell MM, Harig F, et al. Cardiac spiral dual-source CT with high pitch: a feasibility study. *Eur Radiol* 2009; 19: 2357-2362.

[51] Feuchtner G, Goetti R, Plass A, et al. Dual-step prospective ECG-triggered 128-slice dual-source CT for evaluation of coronary arteries and cardiac function without heart rate control: a technical note. *Eur Radiol* 2010; 20: 2092-2099.

[52] Nuyts J, De Man B, Dupont P, et al. Iterative reconstruction for helical CT: a simulation study. *Phys Med Biol* 1998; 43:729–737.

[53] Sun Z, Choo GH, Ng KH. Coronary CT angiography: current status and continuing challenges. *Br J Radiol* 2012; 85; 495-510.

[54] Leipsic J, LaBounty TM, Heilbron B, et al. Estimated radiation dose reduction using adaptive statistical iterative reconstruction in coronary CT angiography: the ERASIR study. *AJR Am J Roentgenol* 2010; 195: 655-660.

[55] Leipsic J, LaBounty TM, Heilbron B, et al. Adaptive statistical iterative reconstruction: assessment of image noise and image quality in coronary CT angiography. *AJR Am J Roentgenol* 2010; 195: 649-654.

[56] Valentin J. The 2007 recommendations of the International Commission on Radiological Protection 103. *Annals of the ICRP* 2007;37:1-332.

[57] Gosling O, Loader R, Venables P, et al: are we under-estimating the dose? A radiation dose study utilising the 2007 ICRP tissue weighting factors and a cardiac specific scan volume. *Clin Radiol* 2010; 65: 1013-1017.

[58] Bongartz G, Golding SJ, Jurik AJ, et al. European guidelines for multislice computed tomography: report EUR 16262 EN 2004. Luxembourg: European Commission, 2004.

[59] Morin RL. Monte Carlo simulation in the radiological sciences. *Boca Raton,* FL: CRC Press; 1988.

[60] Hendel RC, Budoff MJ, Cardella JF, et al. ACC/AHA/ACR/ASE/ASNC /HRS/NASCI/RSNA/SAIP/SCAI/SCCT/SCMR/SIR2008 key data elements and definitions for cardiac imaging. *J Am Coll Cardiol* 2009;53: 91-124.

Chapter 8

Coronary CT Angiography in Coronary Artery Disease: Prospective ECG-Triggering versus Retrospective ECG-Gating

Abstract

With the advent of multislice CT more than a decade ago, coronary CT angiography has demonstrated a huge potential in the less invasive imaging of cardiovascular disease, especially in the diagnosis of coronary artery disease. The diagnostic accuracy of coronary CT angiography has been significantly augmented with the rapid technical developments ranging from the initial 4-slice, to the current 64-slice and 256 and 320-slice CT scanners. This is mainly demonstrated by the improved spatial and temporal resolution when compared to the earlier type of CT scanners.

Traditionally, coronary CT angiography is acquired with retrospective ECG-gating with acquisition of volume data at the cost of increased radiation dose, since data is acquired during the entire cardiac cycle.

Recently, there is an increasing interest in utilising prospective ECG-triggering in cardiac imaging with latest multislice CT scanners (64-slice and beyond) with significant reduction of radiation dose when compared to the retrospectively ECG-gated protocol.

However, there is some debate as to the diagnostic value of prospectively ECG-triggered coronary CT angiography in the diagnosis of coronary artery disease, despite its advantage of lowering the radiation dose.

This chapter will provide an overview of the diagnostic performance of retrospective ECG-gating versus prospective ECG-triggering in the diagnosis of coronary artery disease; highlight the potential applications of prospective ECG-triggering, and explore the future directions of coronary CT angiography in cardiac imaging.

Keywords: Coronary CT angiography, coronary artery disease, diagnostic accuracy, prospective ECG-triggering, radiation dose, retrospective gating

8.1. Introduction

Coronary artery disease (CAD) is the leading cause of death in advanced countries and its prevalence is increasing in developing countries. Invasive coronary angiography is still regarded as the standard of reference for diagnosis of CAD, due to the advantage of superior spatial resolution and temporal resolution. Despite its cost, inconvenience to patients, and a small but distinct procedure-related morbidity (1.5%) and mortality (0.2%) rate, more than one million invasive diagnostic coronary angiography procedures are performed annually in the United States alone. Similarly, CAD is the single most important cause of death in Australia and New Zealand. Every year, billions of dollars have been spent in the treatment of coronary artery disease ($3.9 billion direct spending in Australia 1993-94 according to Australian Institute of Health and Welfare, 2003). Given the invasiveness of coronary angiography and potential danger of having a small risk of serious complications (arrhythmia, stroke, coronary artery dissection and death), a non-invasive technique for imaging of the coronary artery disease is highly desirable.

Imaging of the heart and coronary artery branches has always been technically challenging when compared to the non-cardiac imaging due to the heart's continuous movement. Over the last decade, great strides have been made in the field of cardiac imaging as non-invasive coronary imaging modalities have undergone rapid developments [1-4]. Initially, electron-beam CT was found valuable in coronary calcium scoring as coronary calcum score is a highly sensitive marker with increased prognostic value compared with conventional cardiovascular risk factors for determining the atherosclerotic disease. However, the application of electron-beam CT in the diagnosis of CAD was restricted to a greater extent due to limited spatial resolution [2]. Magnetic resonance imaging (MRI) shows promising results as reported in some studies [3, 4], however, the imaging protocols are variable based on the MRI vendor and software availability which prevents it from being widely used. Imaging of the heart and coronary arteries has become clinically practicable with high diagnostic accuracy achieved, with the introduction of multislice CT and development of electrocardiography-synchronized scanning and reconstruction techniques.

Multislice CT represents technical evolution in cardiac imaging when 4-slice CT scanner was first introduced into the clinical practice in 1998, and this development leads to the widespread application of coronary CT angiography in the diagnosis of CAD [1]. Diagnostic accuracy of coronary CT angiography has been significantly improved with the development of scanning techniques, which are demonstrated by the emergence of 16-, 64-slice and recent models of 256-and 320-slice CT scanners [5-8]. Traditionally, coronary CT angiography was performed with retrospective ECG-gating with high diagnostic accuracy reported for the detection of CAD, however, this is achieved at the cost of high radiation dose since images are acquired with helical scan during the entire cardiac cycle, while only a portion of the data is used for final image reconstruction. Prospective ECG-triggering with axial non-helical scan was used a long time ago with electron-beam CT for calcium scoring. However, in early CT studies of the coronary arteries, the retrospective approach was favoured (and is still widely regarded) as the method of choice to achieve high image quality, especially when patient factors are not favourable for optimal image quality (e.g. arrythmias, high heart rate, etc). The main drawback of the retrospective approach is the relatively higher dose penalty and this has brought back into favour the prospective ECG-triggering.

Recently, prospective ECG-triggering was introduced for coronary CT angiography, and this imaging protocol is increasingly being reported in the literature, despite sufficient evidence is still needed to verify its diagnostic value. This chapter will provide an overview of the diagnostic accuracy of retrospectively ECG-gated CT angiography versus prospectively ECG-triggered coronary CT angiography; the potential applications of prospectively ECG-triggered coronary CT angiography, and highlight some future directions of coronary CT angiography in cardiac imaging.

8.2. Diagnostic Value of Retrospectively ECG-Gated Coronary CT Angiography

The feasibility of coronary CT angiography was initially demonstrated with 4-slice CT using retrospectively ECG-gated technique. Volumetric CT data is acquired throughout the entire cardiac cycle during simultaneous recording of the ECG signal. Subsequently, data from specific periods of the cardiac cycle (most commonly at late diastolic phase) is reconstructed by retrospective referencing to the ECG signal with the aim of generating images with the least motion artefacts. Over the last decade a great deal of interest has been focused on imaging and diagnosis of CAD with multislice CT due to its less invasive nature and fast scanning technique with extended z-axis coverage when compared to single-slice CT. Earlier studies with 4-slice CT showed moderate diagnostic accuracy with pooled sensitivity and specificity of 78% and 93%, respectively [9]. However, image quality was suboptimal in many cases with 4-slice CT due to limited spatial and temporal resolution, and the unassessable segments could be as high as more than 30% in studies performed 4-slice coronary CT angiography [9]. With the introduction of 16-slice CT, image quality in coronary CT angiography has become more consistent with improved results achieved. Studies that used 16-slice CT with acquisition and gantry rotation times of <400 ms have reported sensitivities between 83% and 98% and specificities between 96% and 98% [10-13].

Shorter examination times are possible with further improved diagnostic accuracy with 64-slice CT owing to improved spatial and temporal resolution compared with 16-slice CT. Acquisition of isotropic volume data are made available with 64-slice CT, thus detection of main and side coronary artery branches is improved when compared to earlier types of multislice CT scanners. Several meta-analyses of 64-slice CT studies reported sensitivities of 93% and specificities of 96% (in 6 studies) [14], sensitivities of 97% and specificities of 88% (in 15 studies) [15], and sensitivities of 86% and specificities of 96% (in 19 studies) [16]. These studies concluded that coronary CT angiography, especially with 64-or more slice CT has high diagnostic accuracy for detection of CAD and could be used as an effective alternative to invasive coronary angiography in selected patients.

In 2006, the first dual-source CT (DSCT) scanner was introduced [17]. With the coupling of two X-ray tubes mounted at 90° to each other in a single gantry, the rotation time was shortened, temporal resolution was doubled (83 ms with DSCT vs 165 ms with single-source 64-slice CT), and diagnostic images are still able to be achieved in patients with high heart rate. Studies performed with DSCT showed promising results with high diagnostic accuracy for detection of CAD, and most importantly the image quality is independent of heart rate [18-20]. Leber *et al* [18] in their early study reported DSCT had high diagnostic accuracy for detection of coronary stenoses and image quality was independent of heart rate. The benefit of improved temporal resolution with DSCT is evident with supporting evidence by later studies further confirming its improved accuracy, with heart rate having no significant effect on image quality and diagnostic accuracy [18-21]. Rixe *et al* concluded that high diagnostic accuracy (99% and 92% at segment-based and patient-based analysis, respectively) was achieved even at high heart rates [21]. Heart-rate independent image quality with DSCT represents another milestone in cardiac imaging and it could be used as a reliable alternative to invasive coronary angiography for detection of CAD in patients with high heart rates. A systematic analysis of the diagnostic performance of DSCT coronary angiography has been provided in Chapter 5 with high diagnostic accuracy achieved, and most importantly, the diagnostic performance of DSCT coronary angiography remains high in the presence of high heart rates.

Further technical developments of multislice CT scanners, such as the emergence of wide-area detector CT enabled greater coverage per gantry rotation. Expansion of multislice CT systems from a 64-slice to 128-, 256- and 320-slice system has allowed for the accurate assessment of stenosis severity and atherosclerotic plaque composition, or even the acquisition of whole-heart coverage in one gantry rotation [7, 8, 22-25]. Studies performed with 128- and 256-slice CT demonstrated the ability of coronary CT angiography for quantification of coronary lumen stenosis and assessment of plaque morphology and distribution in the coronary arteries [22, 23]. With 320-slice CT, 16 cm of longitudinal coverage (64-slice CT can only achieve up to 4 cm z-axis coverage, depending upon the detector array width) can be obtained in a single heartbeat, with excellent image quality and demonstration of the entire coronary arterial tree. As shown in Chapter 6, 320-slice coronary CT angiography has high diagnostic accuracy, even in patients with high heart rate or atrial fibrillation [24, 25].

While satisfactory results have been achieved with the retrospectively ECG-gated coronary CT angiography through continuous exposure in a low-helical pitch (0.2-0.4) resulting in multiple overlapping regions of X-ray exposure, the downside is the relatively high effective radiation doses. The radiation dose associated with retrospective ECG-gating is gradually increased with the increased number of detector rows and reduction of detector size [26]. Thus, 4-slice CT scanners have lower dose than 16-slice scanners. Similarly 16-slice scanners have lower doses than 64-slice, and subsequently doses from 64-slice will be lower than those acquired with 256- and 320- slice scanners. Therefore, various strategies have been undertaken to reduce the radiation dose while using coronary CT angiography in cardiac imaging, and prospective ECG-triggering is by far the most effective and significant technique to reduce radiation dose.

8.3. Diagnostic Applications of Prospectively ECG-Triggered Coronary CT Angiography

Prospective ECG-triggering utilizes the same technique as that used in electron-beam CT which is defined as the step-and-shoot method. It is mainly used for quantification of calcium burden, but recently it is increasingly used for coronary CT angiography examinations. The scan is performed in a non-helical way with acquisition of a series of axial images instead of volumetric data. Unlike retrospective gating, prospective ECG- triggering allows for acquisition of data by selectively turning the X-ray tube on only in the selected phase, triggered by the ECG signal, and turning off during the rest of R-R cycle. This is also referred to sequential or step-and-shoot acquisition with prospective triggering and the effective pitch is 1.0. The main advantage of this scanning protocol is the lower radiation dose as X-ray exposure only takes place during the selected cardiac phase rather than throughout the entire cardiac cycle. Therefore, a significant reduction of radiation dose can be expected from prospective ECG-triggering, which is the most attractive advantage of this scanning protocol compared to retrospective ECG-gating.

Recent technical developments of multislice CT imaging technique allows for prospective ECG-triggering to be performed in a single heartbeat with helical scan [27, 28]. Rybicki *et al* in their initial study showed that diagnostic images acquired with prospectively ECG-triggered 320-slice CT angiography were achieved in more than 90% of patients with reduction of radiation dose [8]. In addition to the reduction of motion artefacts, functional assessment of the heart can also be achieved with 320-slice CT since the scan is performed in a single heartbeat [27].

Use of prospective ECG-triggering with 64-slice or DSCT has been reported to reduce the effective radiation dose by up to 90% when compared to retrospectively ECG-gated technique [29-39]. In 2006, Hsieh *et al* [29] first described the step-and-shoot prospectively ECG-triggered protocol for imaging coronary artery disease. They claimed that patient dose could be reduced by at least 50% when compared to the standard retrospectively ECG-gated protocol without compromising image quality. Afterwards, Husmann *et al* [30] in their first clinical experience demonstrated the feasibility of prospective ECG-triggering with low dose results. Diagnostic image quality was achieved in 93% of 41 patients with suspected or proved CAD with very low mean effective dose of 2.1 mSv (1.1-3.0 mSv), when heart rate was less than 63 beats per minute (bpm). This contrasts significantly to the higher radiation dose arising from previous retrospectively ECG-gated coronary CT angiography (up to 21 mSv) [40, 41]. It must be noted that such a high radiation dose results from coronary CT angiography without using ECG-based tube current modulation. The mean effective doses were reduced to less than 10 mSv for 64-slice coronary CT angiography performed with ECG-based tube current modulation [42, 43], although it is still higher than those from prospectively triggered protocols.

Studies comparing prospective triggering and retrospective gating further confirmed the significant reduction of radiation dose with use of prospective triggering protocol. Shuman *et al* in their prospective study compared a group of patients who underwent prospectively triggered coronary CT angiography with another matched group of patients who underwent retrospectively gated protocol. Similar image quality of coronary segments was scored for both groups, but 77% dose reduction was achieved in the prospectively triggered group [31]. This was also confirmed by another two comparative studies performed by Hirai *et al* and Earls *et al* who both showed the similar image quality between prospectively triggered and retrospectively gated protocols, but with dose reduction of 79% and 83% achieved in the prospectively triggered groups [32, 33]. With adequate preparation and patient selection, Earls *et al* concluded that most patients would benefit from prospective triggering with acceptable diagnostic images and significant reduction of effective radiation dose, subsequently reducing the risk of developing radiation-induced malignancies.

Radiation dose can be further reduced with reduction of the tube voltage (kVp), in addition to the tube current modulation which is available in most of the 64-slice scanners. Researchers investigated the prospective triggering with different kVp values, and its effect on radiation dose with promising results achieved. Stolzmann *et al* studied the image quality and radiation dose with DSCT prospective triggering by using different protocols [37]. Their results showed no significant differences in image quality between 100 kVp and 120 kVp protocols, but with significant reduction of radiation dose achieved in 100 kVp protocols (1.2 mSv ± 0.2) compared with 120 kVp protocols (2.6 mSv ± 0.5). Gopal *et al* in their recent study consisting of 149 patients compared prospective triggered and retrospective gated protocols with different kVp groups [35]. A reduction of radiation exposure up to 90% was achieved with use of 100 kVp without compromising image quality. Therefore, there is still room for radiation dose reduction when using the prospectively triggered technique, although more data from multicentres are needed to corroborate these early findings.

It is important to note that while prospectively ECG-triggered coronary CT angiography leads to a significant reduction in effective radiation dose and provides equivalent or improved image quality relative to retrospectively gated images, studies reported in the literature highlight some important limitations to the current multislice CT scanners. The main limitation lies in the fact that image quality is dependent on the heart rate, heart rate variation and body mass index (BMI). Maximum heart rate threshold is between 63-75 bmp for prospectively triggered protocol. When heart rate is greater than 70 bmp, or heart rate variation greater than 10 bmp, or BMI greater than 30 kg/m^2, lower image quality occurs as reported by some studies [36, 37]. All of these limitations indicate that prospectively ECG-triggered coronary CT angiography is limited to patient cohorts strictly defined by the above three factors, thus the prospectively triggered protocol applies only to appropriately selected patients.

Further technical developments in multislice CT technique overcome the above-mentioned limitations with the emergence of new generation of multislice CT techniques such as 256- and 320-slice CT scanners. Longer z-axis coverage available with 256- and 320-slice scanners ranging from 12.8 cm to 16 cm in one gantry rotation permits full cardiac coverage in one gantry rotation with prospective triggering, thus, eliminating the restrictions and limitations associated with 64-slice scanners (maximum z-axis coverage is 4 cm for 64-slice CT) [7, 8]. Huamann *et al* reported that stair-step artefacts in 64-slice coronary CT angiography with prospective ECG-triggering are determined by the BMI and high heart rate variations [44]. Studies using 320-slice CT demonstrated the improvement of prospective triggering with the new generation of CT scanner, eliminating the motion-related artefacts [24, 25]. The majority of patients could be imaged in a single heartbeat with excellent image quality, according to the study performed by Rybicki *et al* [8]. Also, patients with cardiac arrhythmias are no longer excluded from the cardiac CT imaging [25].

8.4. Diagnostic Value of Prospectively ECG-Triggered Coronary CT Angiography

Despite the promising aspect of significant reduction of radiation dose with prospective triggering, there is a lack of sufficient evidence to show the diagnostic value or performance of prospective triggering in the detection of coronary artery disease. Most of the studies currently available in the literature addressed the image quality and reduction of radiation dose when comparing prospectively triggered with retrospectively gated protocols. A direct comparison between prospective triggering and invasive coronary angiography is limited for the diagnosis of coronary stenosis. Scheffel *et al* presented the first report demonstrating the diagnostic performance of low-dose prospective triggering CT for the diagnosis of CAD [37]. Diagnostic accuracy was obtained in patients with heart rate less than 70 bmp with prospectively triggered coronary CT angiography with more than 96% in sensitivity and specificity, whether the analysis was segment-based, vessel-based or patient-based. Stolzmann *et al* also reported the high diagnostic accuracy of prospective triggering for diagnosis of CAD with low radiation dose, even in the presence of heavy calcification, despite the fact that increased rate of non-diagnostic segments was observed due to heavy calcification [45]. Further studies comparing prospective triggering with invasive coronary angiography are required to verify the diagnostic value of this rapidly growing CT imaging protocol. Chapter 10 will provide a systematic review and meta-analysis of the diagnostic performance of prospectively ECG-triggered coronary CT angiography.

8.5. Retrospectively Gated versus Prospectively Triggered Coronary CT Angiography

It seems that the current direction of coronary CT angiography in cardiac imaging is moving from the previous retrospective gating to the currently recommended prospective triggering, and this is demonstrated by the increasing reports available in the literature over the last few years. The main driving force for this trend is the reduction of radiation dose, which is the most attractive aspect of prospectively triggered protocol. Certainly this is only made available due to the technical developments of multislice CT technique, especially with the increased temporal resolution. In order to acquire diagnostic quality images, prospectively ECG-triggered coronary CT angiography must be performed with use of 64 or more slice CT scanners. While radiation dose is significantly lower than that acquired with retrospectively ECG-gated coronary CT angiography, the evidence of prospective triggering for diagnosis of coronary artery disease is insufficient at this stage. Thus, it is too early to draw conclusions that prospectively triggered coronary CT angiography can be used as a reliable alternative to invasive coronary angiography for the diagnosis of coronary artery disease before adequate research evidence is available.

With more research findings available in the literature in the near future, it is expected that coronary CT angiography will be used as a first line technique in cardiac imaging, possibly with prospective triggering replacing the traditional retrospectively gated technique. There is no doubt that coronary CT angiography has entered a new era in cardiac imaging with the advent of 64-, 256- and 320-slice scanners, and its applications in clinical practice will benefit more patients with suspected or proved coronary artery disease. While reduction of radiation dose is important, the most significant aspect of coronary CT angiography is the image quality required for diagnostic purposes. Thus, both of these two factors need to be taken into account when choosing prospectively ECG-triggered coronary CT angiography in the diagnosis of coronary artery disease. The Table 8.1 shows the pros and cons of these two coronary CT angiography protocols. The aim of the following recommendations is to provide some kind of guidance for readers using coronary CT angiography in coronary artery disease:

Table 8.1. Comparison of prospective ECG-triggering and retrospective ECG-gating for diagnosis of coronary artery disease (with 64- or more slice scanners)

Parameters to be compared	Retrospective ECG-gating		Prospective ECG-triggering	
	Pros	Cons	Pros	Cons
Scanning protocols	Axial helical scan allows acquisition of volume data	Exposure takes place during the entire cardiac cycle and only a portion of data is used for reconstruction	Exposure only occurs at a selected cardiac cycle (late diastolic phase)	Axial non-helical scan with most of the manufacturers; Helical scan with 2nd generation of dual-source CT scanner
Image quality (assessable segments)	98-100%	Affected by heavy calcification and high heart rate	95-99%	Affected when heart rate is >70 bpm or irregular
Effect of heart rate	Diagnostic accuracy is high even in higher heart rate; Independent of heart rate with dual-source CT	Diagnostic accuracy slightly decreases with increasing heart rate (70-100 bpm)	High assessable segments and diagnostic value in low and regular heart rate	Limited to heart rate <70 bmp; Limited to regular and stable heart rate
Diagnostic value	High sensitivity and specificity, especially very high negative value	Sensitivity is affected by heavy calcification	High sensitivity and specificity, no significant difference from that of retrospective gating	Limited data available
Prognostic value	High prognostic value in predicting major adverse cardiac events	Most of the studies are conducted at single centres	High prognostic value	Very limited data available in the literature
Radiation dose	Low tube voltage, ECG-controlled tube current modulation could reduce radiation dose	High radiation dose with range of 7.6-31.8 mSv, depending on dose-saving strategies	Significant reduction of with range of 2.1-9.2 mSv, with dose even lower than 1.0 mSv for high-pitch protocol	Radiation dose increased in patients with higher heart rate
Cardiac functional assessment	Available as volume data are acquired	Radiation dose is higher	Functional assessment is only available with 256- or 320-slice CT	Unavailable with 64-slice CT scanners

- With use of 64-slice or dual-source CT, in patients suspected of CAD for whom only the cardiac anatomy or presence or absence of CAD is the main concern, prospective triggering is suggested;
- With use of 64-slice or dual-source CT in patients suspected of CAD, if cardiac functional information will make a meaningful or significant contribution to the CT

assessment or clinical treatment, use of retrospective gating is suggested with additional dose being justified;

- With use of 320-slice CT in cardiac imaging, prospective triggering is recommended since it allows acquisition of dataset in one gantry rotation, thus providing both anatomical assessment and physiological evaluation;
- With use of prospectively triggered protocol, 100 kVp is recommended in patients with BMI less than 30 kg/m^2 for further reduction of the radiation dose;
- Narrowing the phase window width in prospectively triggered protocol is recommended to reduce patient radiation dose in a single heartbeat coronary CT angiography (320-slice CT).

References

[1] Nieman K, Oudkerk M, Rensing BJ, et al. Coronary angiography with multi-slice computed tomography. *Lancet* 2001; 357: 599-603.

[2] O'Malley P, Taylor A, Jackson J, et al. Prognostic value of coronary electron-beam computed tomography for coronary artery disease events in asymptomatic populations. *Am J Cardiol* 2001; 87: 1335-1339.

[3] Danias P, Roussakis A, Ioannidis J. Diagnostic performance of coronary magnetic resonance angiography as compared against conventional x-ray angiography: A meta-analysis. *J Am Coll Cardiol* 2004; 44: 1867-1876.

[4] Finn J, Nael K, Deshpande V, et al. Cardiac MR imaging: State of the technology. *Radiology* 2006; 241: 338-354.

[5] Hoffman U, Moselewski F, Cury RC, et al. Predictive value of 16 slice multidetector spiral computed tomography to detect significant obstructive coronary artery disease in patients at high risk for coronary artery disease. *Circulation* 2004; 110: 2638-2643.

[6] Raff GL, Gallagher MJ, O'Neill WW, et al. Diagnostic accuracy of non-invasive coronary angiography using 64-slice spiral computed tomography. *J Am Coll Cardiol* 2005; 46: 552-557.

[7] Kido T, Kurata A, Higashino H, et al. Cardiac imaging using 256-detecror row four-dimensional CT: preliminary clinical report. *Radiat Med* 2007; 25: 38-44.

[8] Rybicki F, Otero H, Steigner M, et al. Initial evaluation of coronary images from 320-detector row computed tomography. *Int J Cardiovasc Imaging* 2008; 24: 535-546.

[9] Sun Z, Jiang W. Diagnostic value of multislice CT angiography in coronary artery disease: A meta-analysis. *Eur J Radiol* 2006; 60: 279-286.

[10] Nieman K, Cademartiri F, Lemos PA, et al. Reliable noninvasive coronary angiography with fast submillimeter multislice computed tomography. *Circulation* 2002; 106: 2051-2054.

[11] Ropers D, Baum U, Pohle K, et al. Detection of coronary artery stenoses with thin-slice multi-detector row spiral computed tomography and multiplanar reconstruction. *Circulation* 2003; 107: 664-666.

[12] Kuettner A, Trabold T, Schroeder S, et al. Noninvasive detection of coronary artery lesions using 16-detector row multislice spiral computed tomography technology: initial clinical results. *J Am Coll Cardiol* 2004; 44: 1230-1237.

[13] Achenbach S, Ropers S, Pohle FK, et al. Detection of coronary artery stenoses using multi-detector CT with 16x0.75 collimation and 375ms rotation. *Eur Heart J* 2005; 26: 1978-1986.
[14] Vanhoenacker P, Heijenbrok-Kal M, Van Heste R, et al. Diagnostic performance of multidetector CT angiography for assessment of coronary artery disease: meta-analysis. *Radiology* 2007; 244: 419-428.
[15] Sun Z, Lin CH, Davidson R, et al. Diagnostic value of 64-slice CT angiography in coronary artery disease: A systematic review. *Eur J Radiol* 2008; 67: 78-84.
[16] Abdulla J, Abildstrom Z, Gotzsche O, et al. 64-multislice detector computed tomography coronary angiography as potential alternative to conventional coronary angiography: a systematic review and meta-analysis. *Eur Heart J* 2007; 28: 3042-3050.
[17] Flohr TG, McCollough CH, Bruder H, et al. First performance evaluation of a dual source CT (DSCT) system. *Eur Radiol* 2006; 16: 256-268.
[18] Leber AW, Johnson T, Becker A, et al. Diagnostic accuracy of dual-source multi-slice CT coronary angiography in patients with an intermediate pretest likelihood for coronary artery disease. *Eur Heart J* 2007; 28: 2354-2360.
[19] Brodoefel H, Burgstahler C, Tsiflikas I, et al. Dual-source CT: Effect of heart rate, heart rate variability, and calcification on image quality and diagnostic accuracy. *Radiology* 2008; 247: 346-355.
[20] Johnson T, Nikolaou K, Busch S, et al. Diagnostic accuracy of dual-source computed tomography in the diagnosis of coronary artery disease. *Invest Radiol* 2007; 42: 484-491.
[21] Rixe J, Rolf A, Conradi G, et al. Detection of relevant coronary artery disease using dual-source computed tomography in a high probability patient series: comparison with invasive angiography. *Circ J* 2009; 73: 316-322.
[22] Lazoura O, Vlychou M, Vassiou K, et al. 128-detetor-row computed tomography coronary angiography assessing differences in morphology and distribution of atherosclerotic plaques between patients with and without pre-test probability of significant coronary artery disease. *Eur J Radiol* 2011; 77: 123-130.
[23] Mizuno N, Funabashi N, Imada M, Tsunoo T, Endo M, Komuro I. Utility of 256-slice cone beam tomography for real four-dimensional volumetric analysis without electrocardiogram gated acquisition. *Int J Cardiol* 2007; 120:262-267.
[24] Dewey M, Deissenrieder ZF, Laule M, Dubel JP, Schlattmann P, Knebel F, et al. Noninvasive coronary angiography by 320-row computed tomography with lower radiation exposure and maintained diagnostic accuracy: comparison of results with cardiac catheterization in a head-to-head pilot investigation. *Circulation* 2009;120: 867-875.
[25] Pasricha SS, Nandurkar D, Seneviratne SK, Cameron JD, Crossett M, Schneider-Kolsky, et al. Image quality of coronary 320-MDCT in patients with atrial fibrillation: Initial experience. *AJR Am J Roentgenol* 2009; 193: 1514-1521.
[26] Sabarudin A, Sun Z, Ng KH. A systematic review of radiation dose associated with different generations of multidetector CT coronary angiography. *J Med Imaging Radiat Oncol* 2012; 56: 5-17.
[27] Steigner ML, Otero HJ, Cai T, et al. Narrowing the phase window width in prospectively ECG-gated single heart beat 320-detector row coronary CT angiography. *Int J Cardiovasc Imaging* 2009; 25: 85-90.

[28] Kitagawa K, Lardo AC, Lima JAC, George RT. Prospective ECG-gated 320 row detector computed tomography: implications for CT angiography and perfusion imaging. *Int J Cardiovasc Imaging* 2009; 25: 201-208.
[29] Hsieh J, Londt J, Vass M, et al. Step-and-shoot data acquisition and reconstruction for cardiac X-ray computed tomography. *Med Phys* 2006; 33: 4236-4248.
[30] Husmann L, Valenta I, Gaemperli Q, et al. Feasibility of low-dose coronary CT angiography: first experience with prospective ECG-gating. *Eur Heart J* 2008; 29: 191-197.
[31] Shuman WP, Branch KR, May JM, et al. Prospective versus retrospective ECG gating for 64-detector CT of the coronary arteries: comparison of image quality and patient radiation dose. *Radiology* 2008; 248: 431-437.
[32] Hirai N, Horiguchi J, Fujioka C, et al. Prospective versus retrospective ECG-gated 64-detector coronary CT angiography: assessment of image quality, stenosis, and radiation dose. *Radiology* 2008; 248: 424-430.
[33] Earls J, Urban B, Berman E, et al. Prospectively gated transverse coronary CT angiography versus retrospectively gated helical CT technique: improved image quality and reduced radiation dose. *Radiology* 2008; 246: 742-753.
[34] Earls JP, Schrack EC. Prospectively gated low-dose CCTA: 24 months experience in more than 2000 clinical cases. *Int J Cardiovasc Imaging* 2008; 25: 177-187.
[35] Gopal A, Mao S, Karlsberg D, et al. Radiation reduction with prospective ECG-triggering acquisition using 64-multidetector computed tomographic angiography. *Int J Cardiovasc Imaging* 2009; 25: 405-416.
[36] Gustein A, Wolak A, Lee C, et al. Predicting success of prospective and retrospective gating with dual-source coronary computed tomography angiography: development of selection criteria and initial experience. *J Cardiovasc Comput Tomogr* 2008; 2: 81-90.
[37] Stolzmann P, Leschka S, Scheffel H, et al. Dual-source CT in step-and-shoot mode: non-invasive coronary angiography with low radiation dose. *Radiology* 2008; 249: 71-80.
[38] Scheffel H, Alkadhi H, Leschka S, et al. Low-dose CT coronary angiography in the step-and-shoot mode: diagnostic performance. *Heart* 2008; 94: 1132-1137.
[39] Klass O, Jeltsch M, Feuerlein S, et al. Prospectively gated axial CT coronary angiography: preliminary experiences with a novel low-dose technique. *Eur Radiol* 2009; 19: 829-836.
[40] Ropers D, Rixe J, Anders K et al. Usefulness of multidetector row spiral computed tomography with 64- x 0.6-mm collimation and 330-ms rotation for the noninvasive detection of significant coronary artery stenoses. *Am J Cardiol* 2006; 97(3):343-348.
[41] Mollet NR, Cademartiri F, van Mieghem CA et al. High-resolution spiral computed tomography coronary angiography in patients referred for diagnostic conventional coronary angiography. *Circulation* 2005; 112(15):2318-2323.
[42] Hausleirter J, Meyer T, Hadamitzky M, et al. Radiation dose estimates from cardiac multislice computed tomography in daily practice: impact of different protocols on effective dose estimates. *Circulation* 2006; 123: 1305-1310.
[43] Stolzmann P, Scheffel H, Schertler T, et al. Radiation dose estimates in dual source CT computed tomography coronary angiography. *Eur Radiol* 2008; 18: 592-599.

[44] Huamann L, Herzog BA, Burkhard N, et al. Body physique and heart rate variability determine the occurrence of stair-step artefacts in 64-slice CT coronary angiography with prospective ECG-triggering. *Eur Radiol* 2009; 19: 1698-1703.

[45] Stolzmann P, Scheffel H, Leschka S, et al. Diagnostic accuracy of coronary CT angiography using prospective ECG triggering. *AJR Am J Roentgenol* 2008; 191: 1684-1689.

Chapter 9

Coronary CT Angiography Using Prospective ECG-Triggering: An Effective Alternative to Invasive Coronary Angiography

Abstract

Despite the tremendous contributions of coronary CT angiography to the diagnosis of coronary artery disease, radiation dose associated with coronary CT angiography has raised serious concerns in the literature, as the risk of developing radiation-induced malignancy is not negligible. Various dose-saving strategies have been recommended, with some of them resulting in significant dose reduction. Of these strategies, prospective ECG-triggering represents one of the most effective techniques with resultant effective radiation dose similar to or even lower than that of invasive coronary angiography. Prospectively ECG-triggered coronary CT angiography has been increasingly used in the diagnosis of coronary artery disease due to its high diagnostic accuracy with image quality comparable to that of retrospective ECG-gating, but with significantly reduced radiation dose. Successful performance of prospective ECG-triggering depends on strict selection criteria and careful patient preparation. This chapter provides an overview of the diagnostic applications of coronary CT angiography with use of prospective ECG-triggering with a focus on radiation dose reduction. Diagnostic value and prognostic performance of prospectively ECG-triggered coronary CT angiography in patients with suspected coronary artery disease is discussed. Current status and future directions are briefly highlighted.

Keywords: Coronary artery disease, coronary CT angiography, image quality, prospective ECG-triggering, radiation dose

9.1. Introduction

Over the last decade a great deal of interest has been focused on imaging and diagnosis of coronary artery disease (CAD) using coronary CT angiography due to its less invasive nature and improved diagnostic performance. Moderate to high diagnostic accuracy was achieved with 64- or more slice CT, owing to further technical improvements [1-5]. These studies have indicated that coronary CT angiography has high accuracy for the diagnosis of CAD and could be used as an effective alternative to invasive coronary angiography in selected patients. However, coronary CT angiography has the disadvantage of high radiation dose which raises concerns to both clinicians and manufacturers. This is reflected in the changing research directions from the early research focus on the diagnostic value of coronary CT angiography in CAD to the increasingly reported studies investigating the radiation dose reduction and image quality [6].

Radiation dose is becoming a major issue for coronary CT angiography, since more and more studies are being performed with 64- or more-slice CT in the diagnosis of CAD [7-10]. It is estimated that in daily practice, effective dose of coronary CT angiography may reach up to 40 mSv in female patients if no dose-saving strategies are applied, and this is associated with radiation exposure to breast tissues [11]. The radiation risks associated with coronary CT angiography have become a hot topic of debate in the literature [12-14]. The general view about radiation dose is that CT is associated with a risk of cancer development. Therefore, coronary CT angiography should be performed with dose-saving strategies whenever possible to reduce the radiation dose to patients.

Of various dose-saving strategies used in coronary CT angiography [11, 15, 16], prospectively ECG-triggered scanning protocol represents one of the most promising dose-saving techniques with a significant reduction of radiation dose when compared to the retrospective ECG-gating and invasive coronary angiography [17-19]. Early studies demonstrated the diagnostic feasibility of prospective ECG-triggering and later reports confirmed that diagnostic images are acquired with this new technique while achieving the target of reducing the effective dose by up to 90% [20-23]. It has been reported that the effective dose of prospectively ECG-triggered coronary CT angiography is comparable to or even lower than that of invasive coronary angiography [20-27]. Since prospectively ECG-triggered coronary CT angiography shows promising results in the diagnosis of CAD with resultant very low effective dose, it is expected that more and more studies will be conducted with this technique in cardiovascular imaging. It is essential to develop methods that reduce radiation dose without compromising image quality when choosing coronary CT angiography as the main diagnostic modality in cardiac imaging. The purpose of this chapter is to provide an overview of coronary CT angiography with use of prospective ECG-triggering with a focus on the imaging protocols, diagnostic accuracy, prognostic value and radiation dose when compared to conventional retrospective ECG-gating. Future directions on prospectively ECG-triggered coronary CT angiography are highlighted. This chapter will provide readers with a good understanding of the current status of prospective ECG-triggering in the diagnostic applications of coronary artery disease.

9.2. Prospective ECG-Triggering: Technical Requirements

Prospective ECG-triggering with non-helical scan was used a long time ago with electron-beam CT for calcium scoring; however, it was recommended recently for multislice

CT cardiac imaging, and this imaging protocol is increasingly being reported in the literature due to its resultant very low radiation dose [17-27].

Prospective ECG-triggering uses the partial-scan technique to the motion of the heart, which is defined as the step-and-shoot method, so that scan is triggered by ECG signal instead of spiral CT acquisition. This technique allows data to be acquired in a certain phase of cardiac cycle, preferably in the mid-diastolic phase, when cardiac motion is minimal and at the resting state.

This technique contrasts significantly to the retrospectively ECG-gated coronary CT angiography, which acquires the volume data during spiral scanning at a very low pitch (0.2-0.4) so as to produce volume coverage without gaps in each phase of the cardiac cycle with multiple overlapping regions. Prospective triggering is also referred to as sequential data acquisition with an effective pitch of 1.0. The main advantage of this scanning protocol is the very low radiation dose as the X-ray exposure time is short. Most importantly, this prospectively ECG-triggered method is still accurate in diagnosing coronary artery disease. However, there are some several limitations associated with this protocol.

Firstly, it is limited to heart rate less than 65 beats per minute (bpm). Estimation of the next R-R interval may be incorrect when heart rate changes are present such as arrhythmia [28]. Secondly, ECG-triggered sequential scan is usually restricted to scanning with non-overlapping adjacent slices, or slice increments with only small overlap. The scan time to cover the heart volume is thus directly proportional to the slice increment. Consequently, prospective ECG-triggering puts high demand on the z-axis coverage, therefore, it is normally performed with 64- or more slice scanners. Presence of misalignment due to acquisition of images in 4-5 heart beats to cover the entire heart with 64-slice CT is an example of this limitation (Figure 9.1). This can be overcome with the latest 320-slice CT scanner, which enables coverage of the cardiac volume in a single heartbeat (z-axis coverage is up to 16 cm). Lastly, cardiac images are acquired during only a small portion of the R-R interval as ECG-triggered acquisition targets only a specific phase of the cardiac cycle; thus, functional information about cardiac valve or ventricular wall motion is not available [17, 27].

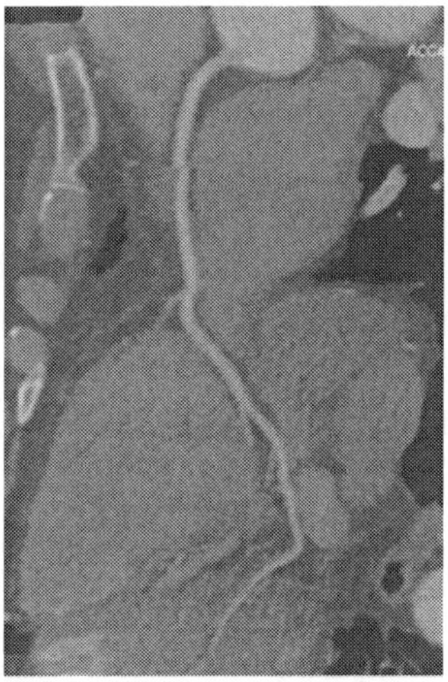

Figure 9.1. Prospectively ECG-triggered coronary CT angiography curved planar reformatted image shows presence of misalignment due to artefacts, affecting visualization of the right coronary artery.

Prospective ECG-triggering can also be performed with high-pitch spiral scan which is a new type of spiral acquisition developed specifically for the second generation of dual-source CT (DSCT) scanner, Siemens Definition Flash. This scanning protocol enables acquisition of 128 slices simultaneously (flying focal spot) [29-31]. The pitch can be increased substantially while still allowing image reconstruction due to dual-source geometry. Overlapping radiation dose is avoided, thus substantially reducing the effective radiation dose to the patient. According to Achenbach and Alkadhi's reports, a very high pitch value (up to 3.4) allowed coverage of the volume of the heart in a very short (approximately 0.260 s), enabling acquisition of complete data in a single cardiac cycle with excellent image quality at a consistent dose lower than 1.0 mSv [29, 31]. Thus, high-pitch spiral coronary CT angiography with prospective triggering is a very attractive approach due to its very low dose.

9.3. Diagnostic Value of Prospective ECG-Triggering at Low Heart Rate

A significant dose reduction has been reported in several studies performed with prospectively ECG-triggered coronary CT angiography [32-34], however, diagnostic value of prospective ECG triggering in the assessment of coronary arteries or CAD has not been systematically studied. Achieving high diagnostic accuracy with prospective ECG-triggering is essential to ensure that this scanning technique can be reliably used as an alternative to high-dose retrospective ECG-gating or invasive coronary angiography in the diagnosis of CAD.

9.3.1. Assessable Coronary Segments and Image Quality

Most of the studies performed with prospectively ECG-triggered coronary CT angiography that are available in the literature focus on the assessment of coronary artery segments and image quality evaluation, in addition to the reduction of radiation dose. The mean assessable segments for prospectively ECG-triggered coronary CT angiography were more than 97%, which are comparable to those for retrospectively ECG-gated scans, according to recent analyses. On average, less than 3% of the coronary segments were reported to be non-diagnostic image quality in prospectively ECG-triggered scans [32, 33].

It is well known that the high-density calcification produces blooming artefacts, which lead to overestimation of the degree of coronary stenosis, thus affecting the assessment of coronary segments and resulting in low positive predictive value. Although it has been reported that the rate of non-diagnostic segments in patients with a higher calcium score was significantly higher than the rate of non-diagnostic segments in patients with a lower calcium score [35], the diagnostic accuracy was not affected in patients with higher calcium loads [36].

Qualitative assessment of image quality was normally performed by a Likert-scale point score system (3 to 5-point ranking scale) in most of the studies, while quantitative assessment of image quality with use of signal-to-noise ratio (SNR) and contrast-to-noise ratio (CNR) was only reported in a few studies [27]. Although image noise (standard deviation) was slightly increased in prospectively ECG-triggered coronary CT angiography when compared to that measured in retrospectively gated scans, there is no significant difference in SNR and CNR between the two groups [27].

9.3.2. Diagnostic Accuracy

Information about diagnostic value of prospectively ECG-triggered coronary CT angiography in CAD is limited, as the majority of currently available studies focus on reduction of radiation dose with acceptable diagnostic images. Two meta-analyses of studies on the use of prospectively ECG-triggered 64-or more slice coronary CT angiography reported that the mean patient-based sensitivities and specificities ranged from 99% to 100%, and 89% to 91%, respectively [36, 37]. The vessel- and segment-based estimates showed lower sensitivities and higher specificities, which ranged from 95% to 97% and 93% to 95%; 91% to 92% and 96% to 97%, respectively. Early evidence indicates that coronary CT angiography with prospective ECG-triggering has high sensitivity and good specificity for the diagnosis of significant CAD. The very high negative predictive value of prospectively ECG-triggered coronary CT angiography with low radiation dose suggests that this imaging technique can be used as a reliable test for ruling out CAD.

Based on the individual studies and meta-analyses, it can be concluded that for the group of patients with a low and regular heart rate (less than 70 bpm) examined to date with coronary CT angiography, use of a prospectively triggered scan has not been shown to change patient-based, vessel-based and segment-based sensitivity or specificity when compared to the existing data for retrospectively gated exams [1-5].

9.4. Diagnostic Value of Prospective ECG-Triggering at High Heart Rate

Although prospectively ECG-triggered coronary CT angiography has high diagnostic accuracy in patients with heart rates below 65 bpm, and radiation dose is low [36, 37], this technique is considered unsuitable for 64-slice and dual-source CT when scanning patients with heart rates more than 70 bpm or significant heart rate variability (e.g. arrhythmia) [38, 39]. For higher heart rates, exposure windows are generally expanded to cover both the systolic and diastolic duration to preserve optimal intervals; however, this comes at the cost of a higher radiation dose [10]. The introduction of 320-slice CT enables whole heart coverage within one heartbeat without requiring table movement, thus, optimal reconstruction intervals could be achieved in patients with higher heart rates using prospective ECG-triggering, while radiation dose is estimated to be lower with high diagnostic accuracy.

Sun *et al* in their study consisting of 47 patients with a mean heart rate of 74.8 bpm reported that prospectively ECG-triggered 320-slice coronary CT angiography had diagnostic sensitivity of 98% and specificity of 99.2%, according to per-segment analysis [40]. In the presence of higher heart rates, image quality was still satisfactory for diagnosis, while the radiation dose was increased from 3.2 mSv when heart rate was less than 70 bpm to 10.2 mSv with heart rate more than 90 bpm. Xu *et al* further confirmed the diagnostic accuracy of 320-

slice coronary CT angiography in 37 patients with persistent atrial fibrillation [41]. The mean heart rate was 88.4 bpm in their prospective group, but 320-slice coronary CT angiography still demonstrated the feasibility in patients with atrial fibrillation, depicting 96.8% diagnostic coronary segments. The sensitivity and specificity of 320-slice CT coronary angiography in the diagnosis of coronary stenosis was more than 90%, either on a per-patient, or per-vessel, or per-segment basis, indicating the high diagnostic performance of prospectively ECG-triggered coronary CT angiography. However, a much higher radiation dose is the main side effect in most patients with atrial fibrillation or premature heart beats due to use of multiple heartbeats for image acquisition [41, 42]. Therefore, dose-reduction strategies, such as lowering tube voltage and adjusting tube current must be implemented to reduce radiation exposure while maintaining diagnostic image quality in this group of patients [41].

9.5. Prognostic Value of Prospective ECG-Triggering

The anatomy-based approach is a well-established method for risk stratification of patients as demonstrated by invasive coronary angiography, which clearly delineates the severity and extent of significant coronary stenosis. High risk coronary anatomy (three-vessel CAD, stenosis of left main coronary artery) is directly related to poorer outcome [43-45], while normal coronary artery is associated with an excellent prognosis [46]. Despite many reports showing the prognostic value of coronary calcifications detected on non-enhanced CT scans, it is not until very recently that the prognostic value of coronary CT angiography has been made clear.

Findings of coronary CT angiography based on a single center experience have been closely associated with the future cardiac events, with 0% or 1% cardiac events being reported in patients with normal cardiac CT or mild coronary artery disease, and up to 30% in patients with one or more vessel obstructive CAD [47-49]. Recently, Abdulla *et al* conducted a meta-analysis of 10 relatively large studies evaluating the prognostic value of 64-slice CT angiography [50]. The meta-analysis showed that cumulative cardiac event rates over a mean follow-up of 21 months were 0.5% in patients with normal coronary CT angiography, 3.5% in those with non-obstructive CAD and 16% in patients with obstructive CAD by 64-slice CT angiography. Compared to a normal coronary CT angiography, non-obstructive CAD was associated with a significant increased risk of major adverse cardiac events, while obstructive CAD was associated with a greatly increased further significant risk.

As mentioned in previous sections, prospectively ECG-triggered coronary CT angiography has demonstrated high diagnostic accuracy in the diagnosis of coronary artery disease, however, its predictive value has not been established. Buechel *et al* in their pioneer study demonstrated the excellent prognostic value of prospectively ECG-triggered coronary CT angiography [51]. Their results showed that coronary CT angiography served as an excellent predictor of even-free survival in the absence of atherosclerotic lesions, while in patients with obstructive lesions, a significant reduction in event-free survival was observed. A 0% of first-year event rate (major adverse cardiac events) was found for patients without any evidence of atherosclerosis, 3% for patients with non-obstructive lesions and 26% for patients with obstructive lesions. Furthermore, the mean effective radiation dose of prospectively ECG-triggered coronary CT angiography in their study was less than 2 mSv. Further studies, particularly, with long-term follow-up are needed to confirm the prognostic value of this low-dose coronary CT angiography.

9.6. Radiation Dose of Prospective ECG-Triggering

Prospective ECG-triggering is associated with lower radiation doses than retrospective gating since in the former case data acquisition is limited to a predicted imaging window of interest. In prospective acquisition, X-ray exposure takes place during one quiescent cardiac phase, most commonly corresponding to ventricular diastasis (usually at the 75% of R-R interval). Thus, single-phase acquisition using prospective triggering depends on accurate prediction of the cardiac phases with minimal cardiac motion. This is feasible with the use of the ECG when the cardiac rhythm is regular and the heart rate variation is minimal [52].

It is an essential step to control patients' heart rate to 70 bpm or lower in coronary CT angiography using prospective ECG-triggering in order to guarantee image quality and low effective dose, as shown in previous studies (Figure 9.2) [17-27]. In patients with high or irregular heart rate, higher radiation dose has been reported in studies due to the use of padding [53-55].

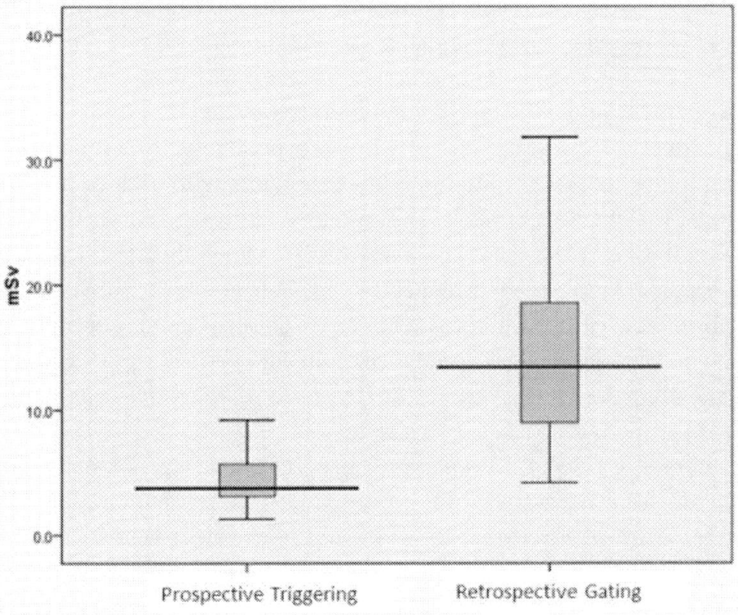

Figure 9.2. Box plot shows the mean effective dose reported in the studies with use of retrospective ECG-gating and prospective ECG-triggering. It is obvious that the radiation dose of prospectively ECG-triggered coronary CT angiography is significantly lower than that of retrospectively gated protocol, according to a systematic review [36]. Horizontal line in each box shows median and top and bottom lines of boxes show interquartile range.

Significant heart rate variation may lead to inaccurate prospective prediction regarding the optimal centring of the imaging window within the expected rest period, and may also result in stair-step artefacts due to misalignment of the imaging windows. To compensate for heart rate variability is to add temporal padding.

The purpose of adding padding (additional surrounding x-ray beam on time) is to provide additional phase information to compensate for variations in heart rate by adding time before and after the centre phase of the acquisition. Padding is described in the range of 0-200 ms and is added to both sides of the center of the acquisition with padding 0 corresponding to a window of 100 ms scanning time and padding 100 corresponding to a window of 200 ms scanning time. Padding is generally used when the heart rates are more than 65 bpm or when there is apparent heart rate variability (heart rate variation is more than 10 bpm) [56]. LaBounty *et al* in their recently published large multicentre study showed that the use of minimal padding was associated with substantial reduction in radiation dose with preserved image interpretability [57].

Use of no or reduced padding should be considered in dose-saving strategies. Freeman *et al* in their prospective study consisting of 2025 patients undergoing prospectively ECG-triggered 64-slice coronary CT angiography reported that the mean effective dose was 2.75 mSv in patients without use of padding, while the mean effective dose was increased to 5.88 mSv in patients studied with padding [54].

Similarly, Hoe and Toh in their study performed with 320-slice CT coronary angiography showed that radiation dose has been significantly increased in patients with heart rate >65 bpm or irregular heart rate when compared to the low heart rate group [55]. The mean effective dose was 5.7 mSv in patients scanned by one-heart beat protocol, but the dose was increased to 13.0 mSv and 17.5 mSv in patients scanned by two- and three-heart beat protocols, respectively. Modification of the prospectively ECG-triggered protocols is necessary to enable further dose reduction in these patients with high or irregular heart rate.

Dual-source CT (DSCT) coronary angiography shows promise in examining patients with different heart rate. Few data are available to show the diagnostic value of DSCT coronary angiography with use of prospective ECG-triggering. Sun *et al* investigated the diagnostic performance of DSCT prospectively ECG-triggered coronary angiography in patients with low to high heart rate, and their results showed no significant difference among low, medium and high heart rate groups in terms of diagnostic image quality, and mean effective dose [53].

Despite encouraging results, patients with irregular heart rate or heart rate more than 90 bpm were excluded from their study due to potential failure or unpredictable image quality (Figs 9.3, 9.4). Xu *et al* explored feasibility of DSCT prospectively ECG-triggered coronary CT angiography in patients with heart rate higher than 70 bpm, and their results indicated that prospective ECG-triggering is feasible in patients with a heart rate between 70 and 110 bpm with excellent depiction of coronary segments and 57% dose reduction compared to the retrospective gating [58].

The second generation of DSCT system with capability of achieving 75 ms temporal resolution could be a promising solution for patients with irregular or high heart rate with use of prospectively ECG-triggered technique.

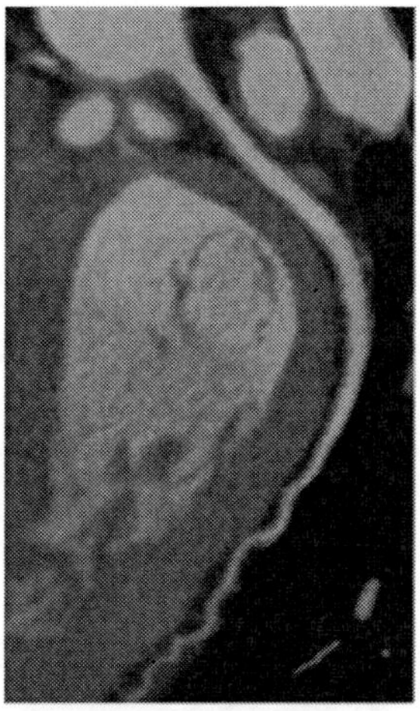

a

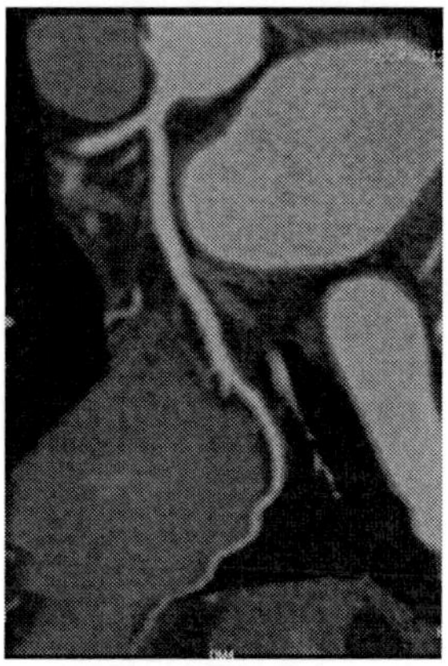

b

Figure 9.3. Prospectively ECG-triggered coronary CT angiography curved planar reformatted images of the right coronary artery (A) and left coronary artery branches (B) with excellent vessel visualization and no artefacts.

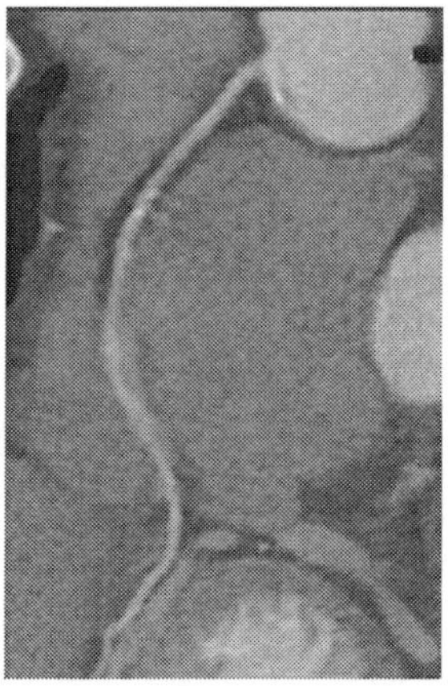

a

Figure 9.4. (Continued).

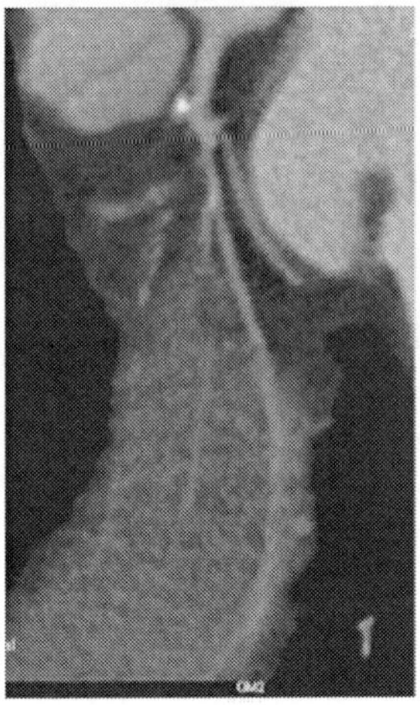

b

Figure 9.4. Prospectively ECG-triggered coronary CT angiography curved planar reformatted images of the right (A) and left coronary arteries (B) with blurred borders due to moderate artefacts.

9.7. Current Status and Future Directions

Current available data indicate that achieving low-dose coronary CT angiography using prospective ECG-triggering is feasible in an everyday population but requires the use of strict exclusion criteria and careful patient preparation [54, 59]. Heart rate control is crucial for performing a successful coronary CT angiography with prospective ECG-triggering with use of either 64- or 128- or 320-slice scanners [20-24, 54, 60-63]. A regular heart rate control of less than 70 bpm is achieved through oral or intravenous administration of β-blockers, and this is conducted in almost all of currently available reports. This may result in the exclusion of patients who do not respond or have known contraindications to β-blockers. DSCT coronary angiography offers potential opportunities for inclusion of patients with different heart rate, although more studies are needed to confirm the diagnostic value and image quality.

The tissue weightings of estimating the effective dose of prospectively ECG-triggered coronary CT angiography are derived from the ICRP (International Commission on Radiological Protection) which focuses on all aspects of protection from ionizing radiation. In 2007, ICRP released the 103 publication updating the 16-year old ICRP 60 dataset, following the latest available scientific information of the biology and physics of radiation exposure, particularly the tissue weighting for breast tissue has increased from 0.05 to 0.12 [64]. The conversion factor used to calculate effective dose from coronary CT angiography has been upgraded from 0.014 to 0.028, thus, doses from coronary CT angiography could be significantly underestimated due to failure of using a cardiac specific conversion factor in the recent ICRP documentation [65, 66]. Gosling *et al* compared the effective dose using the latest ICRP 103 tissue-weighting factors with that calculated with previously published chest conversion factors [65]. Their results showed that the use of chest conversion factors (0.014-0.017) significantly underestimated the effective dose when compared to the dose calculated using the conversion factor of 0.028. A conversion factor of 0.028 would give a better estimation of the effective dose from prospectively ECG-triggered coronary CT angiography. Appropriate conversion factors are needed to accurately estimate effective dose. A conversion factor of 0.014 or 0.017 is commonly used in many cardiac CT studies to estimate the effective dose associated with coronary CT angiography, thus, this could lead to variations in the reported effective dose. As a result, the DLP or CTDIvol is recommended to compare the radiation exposure of coronary CT angiography [56].

Most of the current studies on prospective ECG-triggering are performed by the same expert groups at a single academic center, thus, further studies at multiple centers are needed before widespread implementation of this technique can be recommended.

Conclusion

There is sufficient evidence to confirm that coronary CT angiography with prospective ECG-triggering results in high diagnostic image quality and is associated with a low radiation dose. Prospectively ECG-triggered coronary CT angiography is regarded as a reliable alternative to retrospectively ECG-gated coronary CT angiography in the assessment of coronary arteries in patients with a regular and low heart rate. It is important to note that the current effective doses from prospectively ECG-triggered coronary CT angiography are at the same level or even lower than those acquired from invasive coronary angiography. Therefore, according to the currently available data in the literature, the radiation dose reduction in coronary CT angiography has been very effective and promising. Further studies based on large cohorts with inclusion of patients with different heart rates, and with a focus on the diagnostic and prognostic value are needed to confirm its clinical accuracy.

References

[1] Sun Z, Lin CH, Davidson R, Dong C, Liao Y. Diagnostic value of 64-slice CT angiography in coronary artery disease: A systematic review. *Eur J Radiol* 2008; 67: 78-84.

[2] Vanhoenacker P, Heijenbrok-Kal M, Van Heste R, et al. Diagnostic performance of multidetector CT angiography for assessment of coronary artery disease: meta-analysis. *Radiology* 2007; 244: 419-428

[3] Abdulla J, Abildstrom Z, Gotzsche O, Christensen E, Kober L, Torp-Pedersen C. 64-multislice detector computed tomography coronary angiography as potential alternative to conventional coronary angiography: a systematic review and meta-analysis. *Eur Heart J* 2007; 28: 3042-3050.

[4] Mowatt G, Cook JA, Hillis GS, et al. 64-slice computed tomography angiography in the diagnosis and assessment of coronary artery disease: systematic review and meta-analysis. *Heart* 2008;94: 1386–1393

[5] Stein PD, Yaekoub AY, Matta F, Sostman HD. 64-slice CT for diagnosis of coronary artery disease: a systematic review. *Am J Med* 2008; 121: 715-725.

[6] Sun Z, Ng KH. Coronary computed tomography angiography in coronary artery disease. *World J Cardiol* 2011; 26: 303-310.

[7] Raff GL, Gallagher MJ, O'Neill WW, Goldstein JA. Diagnostic accuracy of non-invasive coronary angiography using 64-slice spiral computed tomography. *J Am Coll Cardiol* 2005, 46:552-557.

[8] Chao SP, Law WY, Kuo CJ, et al. The diagnostic accuracy of 256-row computed tomographic angiography compared with invasive coronary angiography in patients with suspected coronary artery disease. *Eur Heart J* 2010; 31: 1916-1923.

[9] Rybicki F, Otero H, Steigner M, et al. Initial evaluation of coronary images from 320-detector row computed tomography. *Int J Cardiovasc Imaging* 2008; 24:535-546.

[10] Dewey M, Zimmermann E, Deissenrieder ZF, et al. Noninvasive coronary angiography by 320-row computed tomography with lower radiation exposure and maintained diagnostic accuracy: comparison of results with cardiac catheterization in a head-to-head pilot investigation. *Circulation* 2009;120:867-875.

[11] Paul JF, Abada HT. Strategies for reduction of radiation dose in cardiac multislice CT. *Eur Radiol* 2007; 17:2028-2037.

[12] Brenner DJ, Hall EJ. Computed tomography—an increasing source of radiation exposure. *N Engl J Med* 2007; 357(22):2277–2284.

[13] Hausleiter J, Meyer T, Hermann F, et al. Estimated radiation dose associated with cardiac CT angiography. *JAMA* 2009; 301: 500-507.

[14] Raff GL, Chinnaiyan KM, Share DA, et al. Advanced cardiovascular imaging consortium co-Investigators. Radiation dose from cardiac computed tomography before and after implementation of radiation dose-reduction techniques. *JAMA* 2009; 301:2340-2348.

[15] Sun Z, Ng KH. Multislice CT angiography in cardiac imaging. Part III: radiation risk and dose reduction. *Singapore Med J* 2010; 51: 374-380.

[16] Sun Z, Choo GH, Ng KH. Coronary CT angiography: current status and continuing challenges. *Br J Radiol* 2012; 85: 495-510.

[17] Husmann L, Valenta I, Gaemperli O, et al. Feasibility of low-dose coronary CT angiography: first experience with prospective ECG-gating. *Eur Heart J* 2008; 29(2):191–197.

[18] Herzog BA, Wyss CA, Husmann L, et al. First head-to-head comparison of effective radiation dose from low-dose 64-slice CT with prospective ECG-triggering versus invasive coronary angiography. *Heart* 2009; 95: 1656-1661.

[19] Schoenhagen P. Back to the future: coronary CT angiography using prospective ECG triggering. *Eur Heart J* 2008; 29:153–154.

[20] Shuman WP, Branch KR, May JM, et al. Prospective versus retrospective ECG gating for 64-detector CT of the coronary arteries: comparison of image quality and patient radiation dose. *Radiology* 2008; 248(2):431–437.

[21] Pontone G, Andreini D, Bartorelli A, et al. Diagnostic accuracy of coronary computed tomography angiography: A comparison between prospective and retrospective electrocardiogram triggering. *J Am Coll Cardiol* 2009; 54: 346-355.

[22] Huang B, Li J, Law MWM, Zhang J, Shen Y, Khong PL. Radiation dose and cancer risk in retrospectively and prospectively ECG-gated coronary angiography using 64-slice multidetector CT. *Br J Radiol* 2010; 83: 152-158.

[23] Stolzmann P, Goetti R, Baumueller S, et al. Prospective and retrospective ECG-gating for CT coronary angiography perform similarly accurate at low heart rates. *Eur J Radiol* 2011; 79: 85-91.

[24] Hong YJ, Kim SJ, Lee SM, et al. Low-dose coronary computed tomography angiography using prospective ECG-triggering compared to invasive coronary angiography. *Int J Cardiovasc Imaging* 2011; 27: 425-431.
[25] Lu B, Lu JG, Sun ML, et al. Comparison of diagnostic accuracy and radiation dose between prospective triggering and retrospective gated coronary angiography by dual-source computed tomography. *Am J Cardiol* 2011; 107: 1278-1284.
[26] Maruyama T, Takada M, Hasuike T, Yoshikawa A, Namimatsu E, Yoshizumi T. Radiation dose reduction and coronary assessability of prospective electrocardiogram-gated computed tomography coronary angiography: Comparison with retrospective electrocardiogram-gated helical scan. *J Am Coll Cardiol* 2008; 52:1450-1455.
[27] Stolzmann P, Leschka S, Scheffel H, et al. Dual-source CT in step-and-shoot mode: non-invasive coronary angiography with low radiation dose. Radiology 2008; 249:71-80.
[28] Roberts WT, Bax JJ, Davies LC. Cardiac CT and CT coronary angiography: technology and application. *Heart* 2008; 94:781-792.
[29] Achenbach S, Marwan M, Ropers D, et al. Coronary computed tomography angiography with a consistent dose below 1 mSv using prospectively electrocardiogram-triggered high-pitch spiral acquisition. *Eur Heart J* 2010; 31:340-6.
[30] Lell M, Marvan M, Schepis T, et al. Prospectively ECG-triggered high-pitch spiral acquisition for coronary CT angiography using dual source CT: technique and initial experience. *Eur Radiol* 2009; 19:2576-2583.
[31] Alkadhi H, Stolzmann P, Desbiolles L, et al. Low-dose, 128-slice, dual-source CT coronary angiography: accuracy and radiation dose of the high-pitch and the step-and-shoot mode. *Heart* 2010; 96: 933-938.
[32] Hosch W, Heye T, Schulz F, et al. Image quality and radiation dose in 256-slice cardiac computed tomography: comparison of prospective versus retrospective image acquisition protocols. *Eur J Radiol* 2011; 80: 127-135.
[33] Zhang C, Zhang Z, Yan Z, Xu L, Yu W, Wang R. 320-row CT coronary angiography: effect of 100-kV tube voltages on image quality, contrast volume, and radiation dose. *Int J Cardiovasc Imaging* 2011; 27: 1059-1068.
[34] De France T, Dubois E, Gebow D, Ramirez A, Wolf F, Feuchtner GM. Helical prospective ECG-gating in cardiac computed tomography: radiation dose and image quality. *Int J Cardiovasc Imaging* 2010; 26:99-110.
[35] Stolzmann P, Scheffel H, Leschka S, et al. Influence of calcifications on diagnostic accuracy of coronary CT angiography using prospective ECG triggering. *AJR Am J Roentgenol* 2008; 191: 1684-1689.
[36] Sun Z, Ng KH. Diagnostic value of coronary CT angiography with prospective ECG-gating in the diagnosis of coronary artery disease: A systematic review and meta-analysis. *Int J Cardiovasc Imaging* 2012; 28: 2109-2119..
[37] von Ballmoos MW, Haring B, Juillert P, Alkadhi H. Meta-analysis: diagnostic performance of low-radiation-dose coronary computed tomography angiography. *Ann Intern Med* 2011; 154: 413-420.
[38] Earls JP, Berman EL, Urban BA, et al. Prospectively gated transverse coronary CT angiography versus retrospectively gated helical technique: improved image quality and reduced radiation dose. *Radiology* 2008; 246:742–753.

[39] Gutstein A, Wolak A, Lee C, et al. Predicting success of prospective and retrospective gating with dual-source coronary computed tomography angiography: development of selection criteria and initial experience. *J Cardiovasc Comput Tomogr* 2008; 2: 81–90.

[40] Sun G, Li M, Li L, Li G, Jing Z. Study of optimal exposure windows using 320-detector rows dynamic volume CT. *Reports in Medical Imaging* 2010; 3: 115-122.

[41] Xu L, Yang L, Fan Z, Yu W, Lv B, Zhang Z. Diagnostic performance of 320-detector CT coronary angiography in patients with atrial fibrillation: preliminary results. *Eur Radiol* 2011; 21: 936-943.

[42] Zhang T, Bai J, Wang W, Wang D, Shen B. Preliminary study of prospective ECG-gated 320-detector CT coronary angiography in patients with ventricular premature beats. *Plos One* 2012; 7: e38430.

[43] Bell MR, Gersh BJ, Schaff HV, et al. Effect of completeness of revascularization on long-term outcome of patients with three-vessel disease undergoing coronary artery bypass surgery. A report from the Coronary Artery Surgery Study (CASS) Registry. *Circulation* 1992; 86:446–457.

[44] Pepine CJ, Sharaf B, Andrews TC, et al. Relation between clinical, angiographic and ischemic findings at baseline and ischemia-related adverse outcomes at 1 year in the Asymptomatic Cardiac Ischemia Pilot study. ACIP Study Group. *J Am Coll Cardiol* 1997; 29:1483–1489.

[45] Mark DB, Nelson CL, Califf RM, et al. Continuing evolution of therapy for coronary artery disease. Initial results from the era of coronary angioplasty. *Circulation* 1994; 89:2015–2025.

[46] Lichtlen PR, Bargheer K, Wenzlaff P. Long-term prognosis of patients with angina like chest pain and normal coronary angiographic findings. *J Am Coll Cardiol* 1995; 25: 1013–1018.

[47] Gaemperli O, Valenta I, Schepis T, et al. Coronary 64-slice CT angiography predicts outcome in patients with known or suspected coronary artery disease. *Eur Radiol* 2008; 18:1162–1173.

[48] Carrigan TP, Nair D, Schoenhagen P, R.J. et al. Prognostic utility of 64-slice computed tomography in patients with suspected but no documented coronary artery disease. *Eur Heart J* 2009; 30:362-371.

[49] Aldrovandi, E. Maffei, A. Palumbo, S. et al. Prognostic value of computed tomography coronary angiography in patients with suspected coronary artery disease: a 24-month follow-up study. *Eur Radiol* 2009; 19:1653-1660.

[50] Abdulla J, Asferg C, Kofoed KF. Prognostic value of absence or presence of coronary artery disease determined by 64-slice computed tomography coronary angiography: a systematic review and meta-analysis. *Int J Cardiovasc Imaging* 2011; 27: 413-420.

[51] Buechel RR, Pazhenkottil AP, Herzog BA, et al. Prognostic performance of low-dose coronary CT angiography with prospective ECG triggering. *Heart* 2011; 97: 1385-1390.

[52] Efstathopoulos EP, Pantos I, Thalassinou S, et al. Patient radiation doses in cardiac computed tomography: comparison of published results with prospective and retrospective acquisition. *Radiat Prot Dosimetry* 2012; 148: 83-91.

[53] Sun M, Lu B, Wu R, et al. Diagnostic accuracy of dual-source CT coronary angiography with prospective ECG-triggering on different heart rate patients. *Eur Radiol* 2011; 21: 1635-1642.

[54] Freeman A, Learner R, Eggleton S, Lambros J, Friedman D. Marked reduction of effective radiation dose in patients undergoing CT coronary angiography using prospective ECG gating. *Heart Lung Circ* 2011; 20: 512-516.

[55] Hoe J, Toh KH. First experience with 320-row multidetector CT coronary angiography scanning with prospective electrocardiogram gating to reduce radiation dose. *J Cardiovasc Comput Tomogr* 2009; 3: 257-261.

[56] Sun Z, Ng KH. Prospective versus retrospective ECG-gated multislice CT coronary angiography: A systematic review of radiation dose and diagnostic accuracy. *Eur J Radiol* 2012; 81: e94-e100.

[57] LaBounty TM, Leipsic J, Min JK, et al. Effect of padding duration on radiation dose and image quality interpretation in prospectively ECG-triggered coronary CT angiography. *AJR Am J Roentgenol* 2010; 194: 933-937.

[58] Xu L, Yang L, Zhang Z, et al. Low-dose adaptive sequential scan for dual-source CT coronary angiography in patients with high heart rate: comparison with retrospective ECG-gating. *Eur J Radiol* 2010; 76: 183-187.

[59] Buechel RP, Husmann L, Herzog BA, et al. Low-dose computed tomography coronary angiography with prospective electrocardiogram triggering: feasibility in a large population. *J Am Coll Cardiol* 2011; 57:332-336.

[60] Hlaihel C, Bloussel L, Cochet H, et al. Dose and image quality comparison between prospectively gated axial and retrospectively gated helical coronary CT angiography. *Br J Radiol* 2011; 84: 51-57.

[61] Feng Q, Yin Y, Hua X, Zhu R, Hua J, Xu J. Prospective ECG-triggering versus low-dose retrospective ECG-gated 128-channel CT coronary angiography: comparison of image quality and radiation dose. *Clin Radiol* 2010; 65: 809-814.

[62] Duarte R, Fernandez G, Castellon D, Costa JC. Prospective coronary CT angiography 128-MDCT versus retrospective 64-MDCT: improved image quality and reduced radiation dose. *HeartLung Circ* 2011; 20: 119-125.

[63] Qin J, Liu L, Meng X, et al. Prospective versus retrospective ECG gating for 320-detector CT of the coronary arteries: comparison of image quality and patient radiation dose. *Clin Imaging* 2011; 35: 193-197.

[64] Valentin J. The 2007 recommendations of the International Commission on Radiological Protection 103. *Annals of the ICRP* 2007; 37: 2-4.

[65] Gosling O, Loader R, Venables P, Rowles N, Morgan-Hughes G, Roobottom C. Cardiac CT: are we under-estimating the dose? A radiation dose study utilising the 2007 ICRP tissue weighting factors and a cardiac specific scan volume. *Clin Radiol* 2010; 65: 1013-1017.

[66] Einstein AJ, Elliston CD, Arai AE, et al. Radiation dose from single-heartbeat coronary CT angiography performed with a 320-detector row volume scanner. *Radiology* 2010; 254:698-706.

Chapter 10

Coronary CT Angiography with Prospective ECG-Triggering in Coronary Artery Disease: A Systematic Review and Meta-Analysis of Diagnostic Value, Image Quality and Radiation Dose

Abstract

The aim of this chapter is to perform a systematic review and meta-analysis of the diagnostic value of prospectively ECG-triggered coronary CT angiography in the diagnosis of coronary artery disease. A search of biomedical databases for English literature was performed to identify studies investigating the diagnostic value of 64- or more slice CT angiography with use of prospective ECG-triggering in the diagnosis of coronary artery disease. Sensitivity, specificity, positive and negative predictive value estimates pooled across studies were tested using a fixed effects model. Seventeen studies met selection criteria for inclusion in the analysis. Pooled estimates and 95% confidence interval (CI) of sensitivity, specificity, positive and negative predictive value of prospectively ECG-triggered coronary CT angiography for diagnosis of significant coronary stenosis were 99% (95% CI: 98%, 100%), 90% (95% CI: 87%, 93%), 93% (95% CI: 91%, 95%) and 99% (95% CI: 97%, 100%), according to the patient-based assessment. The mean value of sensitivity, specificity, positive and negative predictive value of prospectively ECG-triggered coronary CT angiography were 94% (95% CI: 93%, 96%), 94% (95% CI: 93%, 95%), 85% (95% CI: 81%, 90%), and 97% (95% CI: 96%, 99%), according to vessel-based assessment; 91% (95% CI: 90%, 93%), 97% (95% CI: 97%, 98%), 81% (95% CI: 75%, 88%), 99% (95% CI: 98%, 99%), according to segment-based assessment, respectively. The mean effective dose was 2.91 mSv (95% CI: 1.65, 4.16 mSv) for the prospectively ECG-triggered coronary CT angiography. This analysis shows that for a predominantly male population with high disease prevalence the use of coronary CT angiography with prospective ECG triggering has diagnostic efficacy with a reduced radiation exposure.

Keywords: Coronary artery disease, coronary CT angiography, image quality, prospective triggering, radiation dose

10.1. Introduction

Since the introduction of 64- or more-slice CT technology, coronary CT angiography has been increasingly used in the diagnosis of coronary artery disease (CAD) due to its high diagnostic accuracy owing to the improved spatial and temporal resolution [1-4]. The non-invasiveness and high diagnostic accuracy of coronary CT angiography for CAD have led to rapidly increasing numbers of cardiac CT examinations performed worldwide. However, the risk of radiation exposure associated with coronary CT angiography still remains a challenge compared with invasive coronary angiography, given the fact that CT is a high-dose imaging modality [5]. This has raised serious concerns in the medical field due to the possibility for radiation-induced malignancy [6-9].

In response to these concerns, tremendous progress has been made to lower radiation dose for coronary CT angiography, and various strategies have been undertaken to address this issue. These include automatic exposure control, ECG-triggered current modulation, lower kVp settings, adjustments of pitch value and scan range and prospective ECG-triggering [10]. Of these dose-saving strategies, prospectively ECG-triggered protocol represents the most effective approach with a significant reduction of radiation dose when compared to conventional retrospective ECG-gating [10, 11].

Early studies demonstrated the feasibility of prospective ECG-triggering and later reports confirmed that diagnostic images could be acquired with this new technique while achieving reduction of the effective dose by up to 90% [10, 11]. The effective dose of prospectively ECG-triggered coronary CT angiography has been reported to be comparable to or even lower than that of invasive coronary angiography [12, 13]. Most of the studies reported in the literature focus on the assessment of image quality and radiation dose of prospective ECG-triggering with use of 64- or more slice CT in comparison to retrospective ECG-gating, while the information about diagnostic value of prospective ECG-triggering in CAD is limited [12-14]. Since prospectively ECG-triggered coronary CT angiography shows promising results in the diagnosis of CAD with resultant very low effective dose, we would expect that more and more studies will be performed with this technique in the near future. Thus, achieving high diagnostic accuracy with prospective ECG-triggering is essential to ensure that it can be reliably used as an alternative to high-dose retrospective ECG-gating or invasive coronary angiography in the diagnosis of CAD. The purpose of this chapter was to perform a systematic review and meta-analysis of diagnostic value of coronary CT angiography with use of prospective ECG-triggering in the diagnosis of CAD compared to invasive coronary angiography, based on the currently available literature.

10.2. Materials and Methods

10.2.1. Search Methods

We searched MEDLINE/PUBMED and COCHRANE databases from January 2008 to July 2012 for articles studying the diagnostic value of prospective ECG-triggering using 64- or more slice CT angiography in patients with suspected or confirmed CAD. The key words used in searching the references were: multislice CT/coronary angiography with prospective

/ECG-triggering/ECG-gating, diagnostic value of multislice CT/coronary CT angiography with prospective ECG-triggering, coronary CT angiography and prospective triggering/ECG-gating, prospective ECG-triggering/gating in cardiac imaging. The literature search ranged from 2008 to present as prospective ECG-triggering with coronary CT angiography was first reported in the literature in 2008 [15]. In addition, the reference lists of identified articles were checked to obtain additional relevant articles.

10.2.2. Selection Criteria

Prospective and retrospective studies were included if they met all of the following criteria: (a) studies included at least 10 patients with suspected or known CAD and must be performed using 64- or more slice CT prospectively ECG-triggered protocols as a diagnostic tool for evaluation of coronary artery disease, with >50% lumen stenosis defined as the cut-off criterion for significant stenosis; (b) assessment of diagnostic value of prospectively ECG-triggered 64-or more slice CT angiography in CAD must be addressed at either patient-based, or vessel-based or segment-based analysis when compared to invasive coronary angiography in terms of sensitivity, specificity, positive predictive value (PPV) and negative predictive value (NPV); (c) the absolute number of true positive, true negative, false positive and false negative results of prospectively ECG-triggered coronary CT angiography were available or could be derived from the available data; (d) effective dose of prospectively ECG-triggered protocols was reported in each study. Exclusion criteria were: patients after treatment of coronary stenting or coronary artery bypass grafts or percutaneous coronary intervention. When multiple reports from a single center were published, all reports were reviewed to obtain the most complete information, but studies with potential duplicate or overlapping data were excluded from the analysis.

10.2.3. Data Extraction and Quality Assessment

Data were extracted repeatedly based on study design and procedure techniques. The reviewer assessed the retrieved articles for possible inclusion according to the selection criteria. The reviewer looked for the following characteristics in each study: year of publication; number of participants; mean age; mean heart rate, heart rate variability and body mass index (BMI); percentage of male patients and number of patients receiving beta-blockers; type of imaging unit used for coronary CT angiography; effective dose estimated in each group; number of coronary vessels and segments analysed, and diagnostic accuracy of coronary CT angiography in CAD when compared to invasive coronary angiography.

The quality assessment of included studies was performed using an updated quality assessment tool "QUADAS-2" (Quality Assessment of Diagnostic Accuracy Studies) guidelines [16]. This revised tool is a considerable improvement over the original tool as it allows for more transparent rating of bias and applicability of primary diagnostic accuracy studies.

10.2.4. Statistical analysis

All of the data was entered into Meta Disc (V 1.4, Meta Analysis for Diagnostic and Screening Trials) for analysis. Sensitivity, specificity, PPV and NPV estimates for each study were independently combined across studies using a fixed effects model. Between-study heterogeneity of the sensitivity, specificity, PPV and NPV estimates was tested using the Mantel-Haenszel Chi-squared test with n-1 degree of freedom (n is the number of studies). Statistical hypotheses (2-tailed) were tested at the 5% level of significance.

10.3. Results

10.3.1. General Information

Twenty-two studies met the selection criteria and 17 studies (with 19 comparisons) were finally eligible for analysis [17-38]. Two studies were excluded as the actual number of true positive, true negative, false positive and false negative results was not available in these studies [37, 38]. Although two studies were reported from the same research group, patient data were collected differently, thus both of them were included in the analysis [19, 20]. Six studies were reported from the same research group over different study periods with data being cumulatively accrued [17, 18, 27, 29, 34, 35], but only four of them were used in the analysis [17, 18, 27, 29]. Of these four studies that were eligible for analysis, one study looked at the effect of calcium scores on the diagnostic value of prospective ECG-triggering [17]; another study consisted of the largest number of data collection [18]; one study was conducted with use of the second generation of dual-source CT scanner which is different from the other two studies performed with single-source CT [27]; while the remaining study focused on the diagnostic value of prospective ECG-triggering at low heart rates [29]. Another study was also excluded, despite its meeting the selection criterion [36], since the study included 33% of patients treated with coronary stents, which interfered with the diagnostic value of coronary CT angiography in CAD. Therefore, a total of 5 studies were excluded from the analysis. Figure 10.1 is the flow chart showing the search strategy to obtain these references.

10.3.2. Study Characteristics

Overall, 4345 coronary arteries and 15272 coronary segments were examined in 1063 patients included in the 17 studies. Table 10.1 lists patient's characteristics and study details related to prospectively ECG-triggered coronary CT angiography. Seven out of 17 studies were performed with single-source 64-slice CT, four studies were performed with the first generation of dual-source 64-slice CT, four with the second generation of dual-source CT (128-slice with a pitch value of up to 3.4), and the remaining two studies with 320-slice CT. Seventeen studies provided data at the patient level, 15 at the vessel and 14 at the segment level, respectively. On average, 3% of the coronary segments were reported to be non-diagnostic image quality.

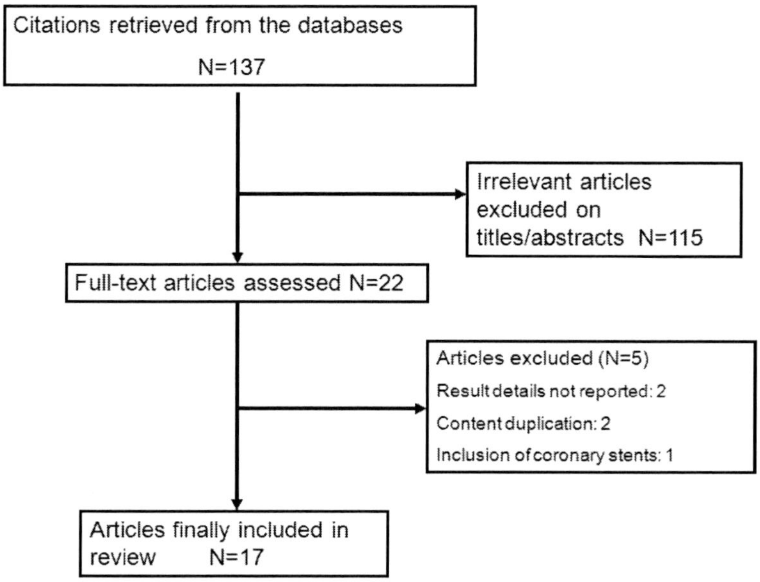

Figure 10.1. Flow chart shows the search strategy used to identify eligible references.

10.3.3. Quality Assessment

Quality assessment of all included studies based on the updated QUADAS-2 is shown in Table 10.2. Overall, the study quality was satisfactory. For all 17 studies, the investigators clearly explained that readers interpreted coronary CT angiography results without any knowledge of the invasive coronary angiography results and vice versa. In addition, operators and readers of coronary CT angiography were unaware of patient history and symptoms in all studies.

10.3.4. Patient Characteristics

The mean prevalence of CAD for study patients was 59.5%, and mean BMI was 26.2 kg/m^2 and the mean age was 62.6 years. The mean heart rate was less than 65 beats per minute (bpm) in 16 studies, while in the remaining study the mean heart rate was 67.7 bmp [30]. Patients were referred for coronary CT angiography and invasive coronary angiography examinations mainly due to the symptom of typical or atypical chest pain in all of the studies. Invasive coronary angiography confirmed that the prevalence of significant CAD (>50% lumen stenosis) was found in more than 50% of patients among 17 studies. Calcium scores were measured in eight studies with nine comparisons, as one study included two groups of patients with different calcium scores [17]. The mean calcium scores were 299.2, indicating the high prevalence of coronary artery disease in these studies. Diagnostic accuracy of coronary CT angiography with use of prospective ECG-triggering was not affected by the presence of heavy calcifications, as reported in one study [17].

Table 10.1. Study characteristics of prospectively ECG-triggered coronary CT angiography in the diagnosis of coronary artery disease

Studies	Year of publication	Detector collimation	No. Patients	No. of cases β blocker %	Mean age (yrs)	No. Male	HR	BMI	Assessable segments (%)	Coronary calcium score	Effective dose (mSv)
Stolzman et al (17)	2008	2x32x0.6	100	21	64.2 ± 6.5	62	60.7 ± 5.4	26.1 ± 2.9	96	316 (108 ± 107/ 1000 ± 547)	2.6±0.8 (3.1±0.5 for 120 kV protocol, 1.7±0.4 for 100 kV protocol)
Scheffel et al (18)	2008	2x 32x0.6	120	47	68.2 ± 8.5	71	59 ± 6	26.2 ± 3.2	98	238	2.5 ± 0.8 (3.0±0.5 for 120 kV protocol, 1.6±0.3 for 100 kV protocol)
Herzog et al (19)	2008	64x0.625	30	67	58.8 ± 9.9	19	55.7 ± 7.9	27.0 ± 4.9	96	NA	2.1 ± 0.7
Herzog et al (20)	2009	64x0.625	42	83	62 ± 8.4	29	55.4 ± 6.2	26.9 ± 4.4	97	NA	2.1 ± 0.7
Pontone et al (21)	2009	64x0.625	80	85	64.8 ± 9.6	70	54.7 ± 5.2	27 ± 3.9	96	375 ± 393	5.7 ± 1.5 (3.8±1.2/0 padding, 5.8±1.8/100 padding, 7.4±3.0/200 padding)
Maruyama et al (22)	2009	64x0.625	76	0	69.9 ± 9.9	47	54.6 ± 6.9	23.6 ± 4.6	96.6	NA	4.3 ± 1.3
Leschka et al (23)	2009	2x64x0.6	35	29	62±8	28	58±3	26.2±3.1	99	NA	0.9±0.1
Dewey et al (24)	2009	320x0.5	30	63	61 ± 10	21	59.6 ± 6.6	NA	NA	384 ± 742	4.2 (3.9 for HR<65, 12.3 for HR>65)
LaBounty et al (25)	2010	64x0.625	45	NA	63 ±12	32	56 ± 10	27 ± 4	98.8	NA	2.6

Studies	Year of publication	Detector collimation	No. Patients	No. of cases β blocker %	Mean age (yrs)	No. Male	HR	BMI	Assessable segments (%)	Coronary calcium score	Effective dose (mSv)
Carrascoca et al (26)	2010	64x0.625	50	92	62.4 ±12.5	33	57.8 ± 5.6	27.7 ± 3.4	97.9	NA	3.4 ± 0.4
Alkadhi et al (27)	2010	2x64x0.6	50	30	62 ± 8	38	58 ± 8	26.4 ± 3.1	98.6	NA	1.4 ± 0.4
Alkadhi et al (27)*	2010	2x64x0.6	50	34	63±8	36	56±10	25.9±2.8	98.9	NA	0.9±0.1
de Graaf et al (28)	2010	320x0.5	64	NA	61 ± 16	34	60 ± 11	26 ± 3	99	184 ± 223	10.8 ± 2.8 (3.9 ± 1.3 at 75% R-R interval, 6.0 ±.3.0 at 65-85% R-R interval)
Husmann et al (29)	2010	64x0.6	61	83	61 ± 11	37	56 ± 7	27 ± 5	NA	481 ± 885	2.1 ± 0.7
Lu et al (30)	2011	2x32x0.6	62	0	57.7 ± 9.7	42	67.7 ±10.5	25.3 ± 3.0	100	254.9±396.3	2.95 ± 1.39
Stolazman et al (31)	2011	2x32x0.6	100	83	68 ± 8	58	58 ± 7	26.3 ± 3.1	98.4	162	2.2 ± 0.4
Achenbach et al (32)	2011	2x64x0.6	50	90	59±12	34	54±6	NA	NA	NA	0.76±0.08
Hu et al (33)	2012	2x64x0.6	103	NA	57±6	73	61	24.5±2.9	98.6	NA	0.9±0.[2a]/1.5±0.3[b]

HR-heart rate, BMI-body mass index, NA- not available.

Alkadhi et al * high pitch mode was applied to this group of patients.

Hu et al [a] Conversion k= 0.017 mSv x mGy x cm^{-1}.

Hu et al [b] Conversion k=0.028 mSv x mGy x cm^{-1}.

Table 10.2. QUADAS-2 results for studies performed with prospectively ECG-triggered coronary CT angiography

Studies	Risk of Bias				Applicability Concerns		
	Patient selection	Index test	Reference standard	Flow and timing	Patient selection	Index test	Reference standard
Stolzman et al (17)	↑	↑	↑	↑	↑	↑	↑
Scheffel et al (18)	↑	↑	↑	↑	↑	↑	↑
Herzog et al (19)	↑↑	↑	↑	?	↑↑	↑	?
Herzog et al (20)	↑	↑	↑	↑	↑	↑	↑
Pontone et al (21)	↑	↑	↑	?	↑	↑	↑
Maruyama et al (22)	↑	↑↑	↑↑	↑	↑	↑↑	↑↑
Leschka et al (23)	↑	↑	↑	↑	↑	↑	↑
Dewey et al (24)	↑	↑	↑	↑	↑	↑	↑
LaBounty et al (25)	↑	↑	↑	↑	↑	↑	↑
Carrascoca et al (26)	↑	↑	↑↑	↑	↑	↑	↑↑
Alkadhi et al (27)	↑	↑	↑	↑	↑	↑	↑
Alkadhi et al (27)*	↑	↑	↑	↑	↑	↑	↑
de Graaf et al (28)	↑↑	↑	↑	↑	↑	↑	↑
Husmann et al (29)	↑	↑	↑	↑	↑	↑	↑
Lu et al (30)	↑↑	↑↑	↑↑	↑	↑↑	↑↑	↑↑
Stolazman et al (31)	↑	↑	↑	↑	↑	↑	↑
Achenbach et al (32)	↑	↑	↑	↑	↑	↑	↑
Hu et al (33)	↑	↑	↑	↑	↑	↑	↑

↑=low risk, ↑↑=high risk, ?= unclear risk
Alkadhi et al * high pitch mode was applied to this group of patients.

10.3.5. Analysis of Study Heterogeneity

We explored sources of clinical and statistical heterogeneity by performing additional analysis of the results. On a segment-based level, a 15-17 segment classification model was used in all of these studies. It is expected that all of the four coronary vessels within any patient should be included in the analysis. Therefore, calculations of sensitivity and specificity involve mixtures (a range of values arising from segments combined with a range of values arising from several vessels, but with variations in contributions, by presence/absence rather than by magnitude, to numerators and denominators). No statistical heterogeneity was found for these analyses (p=0.56-0.72) according to patient-based assessment among these studies, so the pooled estimates across studies were used to demonstrate the diagnostic performance. However, severe heterogeneity/inconsistency was noticed at the vessel-based and segment-based assessment levels (p<0.001), so pooling was avoided, and only the mean values across theses studies were described.

10.3.6. Diagnostic Value

The mean assessable segments for prospectively ECG-triggered coronary CT angiography were 98% (95% CI: 97%, 99%). Pooled estimates and 95% confidence interval (CI) of sensitivity, specificity, PPV and NPV of prospectively ECG-triggered coronary CT angiography for diagnosis of CAD on a patient-based assessment were 99% (95% CI: 98%, 100%), 90% (95% CI: 87%, 93%), 93% (95% CI: 91%, 95%) and 99% (95% CI: 97%, 100%) (Figs 10.2, 10.3).

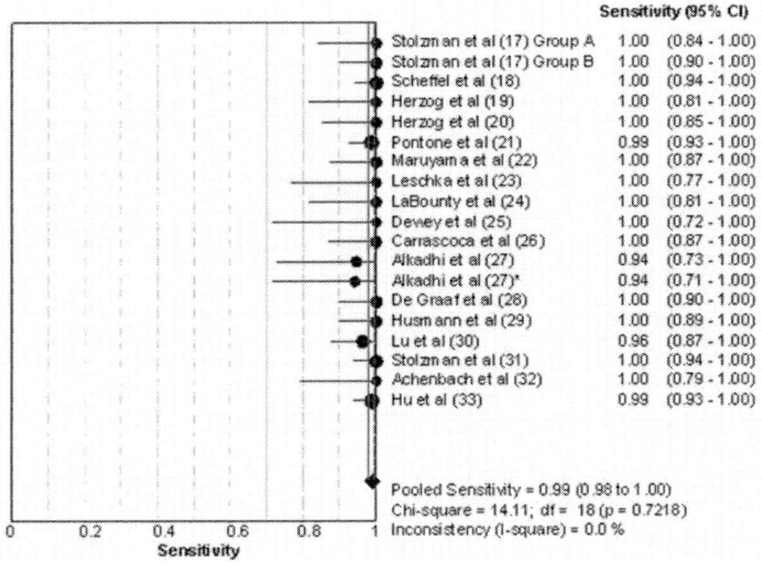

Figure 10.2. Plot and table of pooled sensitivity of prospectively ECG-triggered coronary CT angiography compared to invasive coronary angiography in 17 studies (19 comparisons) based on patient-based assessment. CI-confidence interval. Group A consists of patients with Agatson score less than 316, while Group B consists of patients with Agatston score more than 316. Alkadhi et al (27)'s study involved comparison of two groups with one group undergoing standard prospective triggering, while another group undergoing high-pitch mode.

The mean values of sensitivity, specificity, PPV and NPV were 94% (95% CI: 93%, 96%), 94% (95% CI: 93%, 95%), 85% (95% CI: 81%, 90%), and 97% (95% CI: 96%, 99%), according to vessel-based assessment; 91% (95% CI: 90%, 93%), 97% (95% CI: 97%, 98%), 81% (95% CI: 75%, 88%), 99% (95% CI: 98%, 99%), according to segment-based assessment, respectively.

Diagnostic value of prospective ECG-triggering with inclusion of non-diagnostic segments was reported in two studies [19, 28], however, the analysis of these results was not conducted as inclusion of non-diagnostic segments could make the diagnostic value invalid. In addition to the criterion of 50% coronary stenosis, more than 70% stenosis was also analysed in two studies [24, 33]. The limited data of these two studies did not allow a statistical analysis.

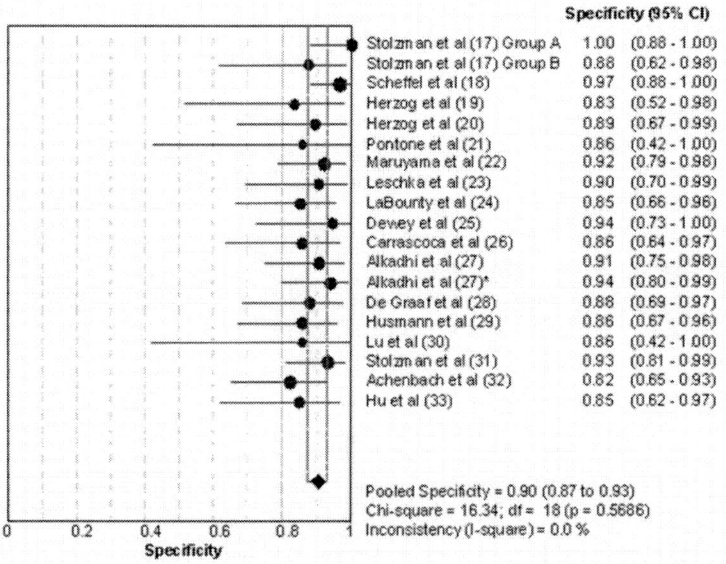

Figure 10.3. Plot and table of pooled specificity of prospectively ECG-triggered coronary CT angiography compared to invasive coronary angiography in 17 studies (19 comparisons) based on patient-based assessment. CI-confidence interval. Group A consists of patients with Agatson score less than 316, while Group B consists of patients with Agatston score more than 316. Alkadhi et al (27)'s study involved comparison of two groups with one group undergoing standard prospective triggering, while another group undergoing high-pitch mode.

10.3.7. Effective Dose

Effective dose was estimated by multiplying the dose length product with a conversion coefficient of 0.014 and 0.017 used in 4 and 13 studies, respectively. The calculation of the effective dose in these studies is based on a method proposed by the European Working Group for Guidelines on Quality Criteria in CT [39], deriving radiation dose estimates from the product of the dose length product and an organ weighting factor for the chest as the investigated anatomic region (k = 0.014 or 0.107 $mSv*mGy^{-1}*cm^{-1}$ averaged between male and female models from Monte Carlo simulations) [40]. In addition to the conversion coefficient of 0.017, a new coefficient of 0.028 $mSv*mGy^{-1}* cm^{-1}$ was used as the coefficient to calculate the effective dose in another study [33]. This was proposed by Gosling and Einstein to reflect the increased weighting factor of the breast during cardiac CT imaging [41-43].

The mean effective dose was 2.91 mSv (95% CI: 1.65, 4.16 mSv) for the prospectively ECG-triggered coronary CT angiography among all of these studies. There were 4 studies performed with the second generation of dual-source CT scanners, with a high-pitch value of up to 3.4 applied in coronary CT angiography. The mean effective dose of the high-pitch prospectively ECG-triggered coronary CT angiography was 0.87 mSv (95% CI: 0.75, 0.98 mSv), and this was significantly lower than that acquired with the conventional prospectively ECG-triggered coronary CT angiography, which was 3.53 mSv (95% CI: 2.03, 5.03 mSv) ($p=0.01$).

A kVp of 100 and 120 was both applied and compared in two studies with use of prospectively ECG-triggered protocol, and a reduction of effective dose by up to 46% was found in the studies scanned with 100 kVp (mean dose 1.65 mSv) when compared to those with 120 kVp (mean dose 3.05 mSv), indicating a further dose reduction of radiation dose with use of lower kVp values in patients with BMI less than 25 kg/m^2.

Padding was applied in one study to manage patients with heart rate variations [21]. The purpose of adding padding is to provide additional phase information to compensate for variations in heart rate by adding time before and after the centre phase of the acquisition. Padding is generally used when the heart rates are more than 60 bpm or when there exists apparent heart rate variability (more than 2 beats/min). Application of padding helps to generate diagnostic images in patients with high heart rate variations, however, this leads to an increase of effective dose by up to 90% when compared to that from without padding groups, as shown in this study.

Discussion

In this analysis, we focused on the diagnostic performance of prospectively ECG-triggered coronary CT angiography for the detection of obstructive coronary artery disease. This systematic review and meta-analysis shows three important findings which are considered valuable from clinical perspectives. Firstly, the mean assessable segments of prospective ECG-triggering are very high (98%), and this indicates a very high value of prospective ECG-triggering for evaluation of coronary arteries. Secondly, the analysis shows that prospectively ECG-triggered coronary CT angiography has a high diagnostic value (>90% for both sensitivity and specificity) in the diagnosis of coronary artery disease in patients with a low heart rate, at all three levels (patient-, vessel and segment-based levels). This indicates that it could be used as a reliable alternative to retrospective ECG-gating and invasive coronary angiography in selected patients. Thirdly, the effective dose associated with prospectively ECG-triggered coronary CT angiography is less than 3.0 mSv, which is comparable to or even lower than that of invasive coronary angiography.

Coronary angiography has been increasingly used in cardiac imaging since 64- and more slice CT shows improved and promising results in the diagnosis of CAD [1-4]. Several meta-analyses of studies on the use of retrospectively ECG-gated 64-slice CT reported mean sensitivities and specificities ranging from 85% to 99%, and 86% to 96%, respectively [44-47]. The mean diagnostic performance reported in this analysis is consistent with those recent reports. The very high specificity and negative predictive value of prospective ECG-triggering allows this technique to be used reliably as an alternative modality for the diagnosis of CAD. Based on this analysis, it can be concluded that for the group of patients examined to date with coronary CT angiography, use of a prospectively triggered exam has not been shown to change patient-based, vessel-based and segment-based sensitivity or specificity when compared to the existing data for retrospectively gated exams.

Despite promising results having been achieved with coronary CT angiography, CT has the disadvantage of high radiation dose, which leads to the concern of radiation-associated risks [6-8]. Of various approaches that have been recommended to reduce the radiation dose of coronary CT angiography, prospective ECG-triggering has been reported to result in a significant reduction of effective dose when compared to retrospective ECG-gating [48, 49]. This analysis is consistent with these reports with regard to the low effective dose resulting from prospective ECG-triggering. With use of prospective ECG-triggering, it is possible to produce diagnostic images with effective dose even lower than that of invasive coronary angiography.

Recently, the second generation of dual-source CT scanners was introduced, providing long detector coverage with use of 128-slice detectors [50-52]. This dual-source CT scanner allows coronary CT angiography to be performed at high pitch values of up to 3.4. In the prospectively ECG-triggered coronary CT angiography with 64- or more slice scanners, the pitch is set at 1.0 to ensure axial scans, while the applicable pitch is limited to values from 0.2 to 0.4 in retrospectively ECG-gated scans to ensure gapless volume coverage of the heart. By combining high pitch and large detector coverage, coronary CT angiography acquisition time is reduced to a quarter of a second, allowing acquisition of the entire heart within a single heartbeat with a temporal resolution of 75 ms. Radiation exposure is inversely proportional to pitch in the ECG-gated spiral CT. Thus, the high-pitch coronary CT angiography is a low radiation dose technique with average values of 1 mSv [12, 13, 53, 54], significantly lower than that of standard retrospectively ECG-gated spiral CT even with use of ECG-controlled tube current modulation. This is confirmed in this analysis as the mean effective dose of high-pitch prospectively ECG-triggered coronary CT angiography is 0.87 mSv and this is significantly lower than that acquired from the low-pitch protocol, while still maintaining high diagnostic accuracy. There are only four studies included in this analysis for assessment of the diagnostic performance of prospectively ECG-triggered coronary CT angiography, since most of the current studies performed with high-pitch mode focus on image quality and radiation dose. Thus further studies are needed to verify its diagnostic value in the detection of coronary stenosis with resultant very low dose.

Appropriate use of lower kVp values (80 or 100 kVp) for coronary CT angiography examinations can further reduce radiation dose without compromising the image quality. Recent studies utilising dual-source CT compared a 100 kVp protocol to the routine 120 kVp for cardiac CT angiography, and demonstrated a dose reduction of 25-54%, with an estimated effective dose as low as 4.4 mSv [55, 56]. With use of a lower kVp in prospective ECG-triggering, a further dose reduction by 46% was achieved with acquisition of diagnostic images with a mean dose of less than 2.0 mSv, as indicated in this analysis. Thus, a combination of prospective ECG-triggering with a low kVp protocol should be recommended in patients with BMI less than 25 kg/m^2, since changing tube voltage needs to be correlated with the patient's BMI.

Some limitations in this analysis should be addressed. Firstly, the publication bias exists and may affect the results as non-English publications were excluded. However, it is reported that language-restriction meta-analyses overestimated the treatment effect by only 2% on average compared with language-inclusive meta-analyses [57]. Secondly, coronary CT angiography was performed in patients referred for invasive coronary angiography, creating a selection bias of patients with a relatively high prevalence of significant CAD. Significant CAD was confirmed in approximately 60% of the patients by coronary angiography in this analysis, indicating the high prevalence of CAD among the patients. Thus, the present diagnostic performance was achieved in an intermediate-to-high prevalence patient population. As a result, the current data (in terms of very high sensitivity and specificity values) may not be directly applicable to patients with a low-to-intermediate prevalence of CAD.

Lastly, effective dose based on a conversion factor is only an estimate. Because the mathematical modelling done to compute organ doses is based on a standard adult (70kg), effective dose estimation can underestimate the risk for children and thin patients and overestimate the risk for obese patients. Therefore, one should remember that the uncertainty associated with the effective dose estimations could vary as much as 40% in some cases. One has to adopt a correction factor when making comparisons with different studies. Although the use of effective dose estimates for assessing the exposure of patients has severe limitations, the effective dose is still widely used as a dose parameter to reflect the radiation risk and compare doses from different diagnostic and therapeutic imaging procedures in different hospitals and countries as well as of different technologies for the same medical examinations.

In conclusion, this systematic review and meta-analysis shows that prospectively ECG-triggered coronary CT angiography has high diagnostic value with a low radiation dose in the diagnosis of obstructive coronary artery disease. The very high specificity and negative predictive value allows it to be used as a reliable alternative to retrospective ECG-gating in patients with a regular and low heart rate.

Acknowledgment

The authors would like to thank Mr Gil Stevenson for his assistance in the statistical analysis of results.

References

[1] Raff GL, Gallagher MJ, O'Neill WW, Goldstein JA. Diagnostic accuracy of non-invasive coronary angiography using 64-slice spiral computed tomography. *J Am Coll Cardiol* 2005; 46:552-557.

[2] Feng Q, Yin Y, Hua X, Zhu R, Hua J, Xu J. Prospective ECG triggering versus low-dose retrospective ECG-gated 128-channel CT coronary angiography: comparison of image quality and radiation dose. *Clin Radiol* 2010; 65: 809-814.

[3] Kitagawa K, Lardo AC, Lima JAC, George RT. Prospective ECG-gated 320 row detector computed tomography: implications for CT angiography and perfusion imaging. *Int J Cardiovasc Imaging* 2009; 25: 201-208.

[4] Ribicki FJ, Otero HJ, Steigner ML, et al. Initial evaluation of coronary images from 320-detector row computed tomography. *Int J Cardiovasc Imaging* 2008; 24: 535-546.

[5] Fazel R, Krumholz HM, Wang YF, et al. Exposure to low-dose ionizing radiation from medical imaging procedures. *N Engl J Med* 2009; 361: 849-857.

[6] Paul JF, Abada HT. Strategies for reduction of radiation dose in cardiac multislice CT. *Eur Radiol* 2007; 17:2028-2037.

[7] Brenner DJ, Hall EJ. Computed tomography—an increasing source of radiation exposure. *N Engl J Med* 2007; 357(22):2277–2284.

[8] Hausleiter J, Meyer T, Hermann F et al. Estimated radiation dose associated with cardiac CT angiography. *JAMA* 2009; 301(5):500–507.

[9] Raff GL, Chinnaiyan KM, Share DA, et al. Radiation dose from cardiac computed tomography before and after implementation of radiation dose-reduction techniques. *JAMA* 2009; 301:2340-2348.

[10] Sun Z, Ng KH. Multislice CT angiography in cardiac imaging. Part III: radiation risk and dose reduction. *Singapore Med J* 2010; 51: 374-380.

[11] Sun Z, Ng KH. Prospective versus retrospective ECG-gated multislice CT coronary angiography: A systematic review of radiation dose and image quality. *Eur J Radiol* 2012; 81: e94-e100.

[12] Achenbach S, Marwan M, Ropers D, et al. Coronary computed tomography angiography with a consistent dose below 1 mSv using prospectively electrocardiogram-triggered high-pitch spiral acquisition. *Eur Heart J* 2010; 31:340-6.

[13] Lell MM, Marvan M, Schepis T, et al. Prospectively ECG-triggered high-pitch spiral acquisition for coronary CT angiography using dual source CT: technique and initial experience. *Eur Radiol* 2009; 19:2576-2583.

[14] von Ballmoos MY, Haring B, Juillert P, Alkadhi H. Meta-analysis: diagnostic performance of low-radiation-dose coronary computed tomography angiography. *Ann Intern Med* 2011; 154: 413-420.

[15] Hsieh J, Londt J, Vass M, Li J, Tang X, Okerlund D. Step-and-shoot data acquisition and reconstruction for cardiac x-ray computed tomography. *Med Phys* 2006; 33:4236–48.

[16] Whiting P, Rutjes AWS, Westwood ME, et al. QUADAS-2: A revised tool for the quality assessment of diagnostic accuracy studies. *Ann Intern Med* 2011; 155: 529-536.

[17] Stolzmann P, Scheffel H, Leschka S, et al. Influence of calcification on diagnostic accuracy of coronary CT angiography using prospective ECG triggering. *AJR Am J Roentgenol* 2008; 191: 1684-1689.

[18] Scheffel H, Alkadhi H, Leschka S, et al. Low-dose CT coronary angiography in the step-and-shoot mode: diagnostic performance. *Heart* 2008; 94: 1132-1137.

[19] Herzog BA, Husmann L, Burkhard N, et al. Accuracy of low-dose computed tomography coronary angiography using prospective electrocardiogram-triggering: first clinical experience. *Eur Heart J* 2008; 29: 3037-3042.

[20] Herzog BA, Wyss CA, Husmann L, et al. First head-to-head comparison of effective radiation dose from low-dose 64-slice CT with prospective ECG-triggering versus invasive coronary angiography. *Heart* 2009; 95: 1656-1661.

[21] Pontone G, Andreini D, Bartoreli A, et al. Diagnostic accuracy of coronary computed tomography angiography: A comparison between prospective and retrospective electrocardiogram triggering. *J Am Coll Cardiol* 2009; 54: 346-355.

[22] Maruyama T, Takada M, Hasuike T, et al. Radiation dose reduction and coronary assessability of prospective electrocardiogram-gated computed tomography coronary angiography: Comparison with retrospective electrocardiogram-gated helical scan. *J Am Coll Cardiol* 2008; 52:1450-1455.

[23] Leschka S, Stolzmann P, Desbiolles L, et al. Diagnostic accuracy of high-pitch dual-source CT for the assessment of coronary stenoses: first experience. *Eur Radiol* 2009; 19: 2896-2903.

[24] Dewey M, Zimmermann E, Deissenrieder F, et al. Noninvasive coronary angiography by 320-row computed tomography with lower radiation exposure and maintained diagnostic accuracy: comparison of results with cardiac catheterization in a head-to-head pilot investigation. *Circulation* 2009; 120: 867-875.

[25] La Bounty TM, Leipsic J, Mancini J, et al. Effect of a standardized radiation dose reduction protocol on diagnostic accuracy of coronary computed tomographic angiography. *Am J Cardiol* 2010; 106: 287-292.

[26] Carrascoca P, Capunay C, Deviggiano A, et al. Accuracy of low-dose prospectively gated axial coronary CT angiography for the assessment of coronary artery stenosis in patients with stable heart rate. *J Cardiovasc Comput Tomogr* 2010; 4: 197-205.

[27] Alkadhi H, Stolzmann P, Desbiolles L, et al. Low-dose, 128-slice, dual-source CT coronary angiography: accuracy and radiation dose of the high-pitch and the step-and-shoot mode. *Heart* 2010; 96: 933-938.

[28] de Graaf FR, Schuijf JD, van Velzen JE, et al. Diagnostic accuracy of 320-row multidetector computed tomography coronary angiography in the non-invasive evaluation of significant coronary artery disease. *Eur Heart J* 2010; 31: 1908-1915.

[29] Husmann L, Herzog BA, Burger IA, et al. Usefulness of additional coronary calcium scoring in the low-dose CT coronary angiography with prospective ECG-triggering. *Acad Radiol* 2010; 17: 201-206.

[30] Lu B, Lu JG, Sun ML, et al. Comparison of diagnostic accuracy and radiation dose between prospective triggering and retrospective gated coronary angiography by dual-source computed tomography. *Am J Cardiol* 2011; 107: 1278-1284.

[31] Stolzmann P, Goetti R, Baumueller S, et al. rospective and retrospective ECG-gating for CT coronary angiography perform similarly accurate at low heart rates. *Eur J Radiol* 2011; 79: 85-91.

[32] Achenbach S, Goroll T, Seltmann M, et al. Detection of coronary artery stenoses by low-dose, prospectively ECG-triggered, high-pitch spiral coronary CT angiography. *JACC Cardiovasc Imaging* 2011; 4: 328-337.

[33] Hu XH, Zheng WL, Wang D, et al. Accuracy of high-pitch prospectively ECG-triggering CT coronary angiography for assessment of stenosis in 103 patients: comparison with invasive coronary angiography. *Clin Radiol* 2012; 67: 1083-1088..

[34] Scheffel H, Stolzmann P, Alkadhi H, et al. Low-dose CT and cardiac MR for the diagnosis of coronary artery disease: accuracy of single and combined approaches. *Int J Cardiovasc Imaging* 2010; 26: 579-590.

[35] Donati OF, Stolzmann P, Desbiolles L, et al. Coronary artery disease: which degree of coronary artery stenosis is indicative of ischemia? *Eur J Radiol* 2011; 80: 120-126.

[36] Chao SP, Law WY, Kuo CJ, et al. The diagnostic accuracy of 256-row computed tomographic angiography compared with invasive coronary angiography in patients with suspected coronary artery disease. *Eur Heart J* 2010; 31: 1916-1923.

[37] Hong YJ, Kim SJ, Lee SM, et al. Low-dose coronary computed tomography angiography using prospective ECG-triggering compared to invasive coronary angiography. *Int J Cardiovasc Imaging* 2011; 27: 425-431.

[38] Korosoglou G, Mueller D, Lehrke S, et al. Quantitative assessment of stenosis severity and atherosclerotic plaque composition using 256-slice computed tomography. *Eur Radiol* 2010; 20: 1841-1850.

[39] Bongartz G, Golding SJ, Jurik AJ, et al. European guidelines for multislice computed tomography: *report EUR 16262 EN.* Luxembourg: European Commission, 2004.

[40] Morin RL. Monte Carlo simulation in the radiological sciences. *Boca Raton,* FL: CRC Press, 1988.

[41] Gosling O, Loader R, Venables P, et al. Cardiac CT: are we underestimating the dose? A radiation dose study utilizing the 2007 ICRP tissue weighting factors and cardiac specific scan volume. *Clin Radiol* 2010;65:1013-1017.

[42] Gosling O, Loader R, Venables P, et al. A comparison of radiation dosesbetween state-of-the-art multislice CT coronary angiography with iterative reconstruction, multislice CT coronary angiography with standard filtered back-projection and invasive diagnostic coronary angiography. *Heart* 2010;96:922-926.

[43] Einstein AJ, Elliston CD, Arai AE, et al. Radiation dose from single-heart beat coronary CT angiography performed with a 320-detector row volume scanner. *Radiology* 2010;254:698-706.

[44] Sun Z, Lin CH, Davidson R, Dong C, Liao Y. Diagnostic value of 64-slice CT angiography in coronary artery disease: A systematic review. *Eur J Radiol* 2008; 67: 78-84.

[45] Abdulla J, Abildstrom Z, Gotzsche O, et al. 64-multislice detector computed tomography coronary angiography as potential alternative to conventional coronary angiography: a systematic review and meta-analysis. *Eur Heart J* 2007; 28: 3042-3050.

[46] Vanhoenacker P, Heijenbrok-Kal M, Van Heste R, et al. Diagnostic performance of multidetector CT angiography for assessment of coronary artery disease: meta-analysis. *Radiology* 2007; 244: 419-428.

[47] Mowatt G, Cook JA, Hillis GS, et al. 64-slice computed tomography angiography in the diagnosis and assessment of coronary artery disease: systematic review and meta-analysis. *Heart* 2008; 94: 1386–1393.

[48] Shuman WP, Branch KR, May JM, et al. Whole-chest 64-MDCT of emergency department patients with nonspecific chest pain: radiation dose and coronary artery image quality with prospective ECG triggering versus retrospective ECG gating. *AJR Am J Roentgenol 2009*; 192: 1662-1667.

[49] Arnoldi E, Johnson TR, Rist C, et al. Adequate image quality with reduced radiation dose in prospectively triggered coronary CTA compared with retrospective techniques. *Eur Radiol* 2009; 19: 2147-2155.

[50] Ertel D, Lell MM, Harig F, et al. Cardiac spiral dual-source CT with high pitch: a feasibility study. *Eur Radiol* 2009; 19:2357–2362.

[51] Goetti R, Baumuller S, Feuchtner G, et al. High pitch dual-source CT angiography of the thoracic and abdominal aorta: is simultaneous coronary artery assessment possible? *AJR Am J Roentgenol* 2010; 194:938–944.

[52] Stolzmann P, Goetti RP, Manrovich-Horvat P, et al. Predictors of image quality in high-pitch coronary CT angiography. *AJR Am J Roentgenol* 2011; 197: 851-858.

[53] Sommer WH, Albrecht E, Bamberg F, et al. Feasibility and radiation dose of high-pitch acquisition protocols in patients undergoing dual-source cardiac CT. *AJR Am J Roentgenol* 2010; 195: 1306-1312.

[54] Scharf M, Bink R, May MS, et al. High-pitch thoracic CT with simultaneous assessment of coronary arteries. *JACC Cardiovasc Imaging* 2011; 4: 602-609.

[55] Pflederer T, Rudofsky L, Ropers D, et al. Image quality in a low radiation exposure protocol for retrospectively ECG-gated coronary CT angiography. *AJR Am J Roentgenol* 2009; 192:1045-1050.

[56] Leschka S, Stolzmann P, Schmid F, et al. Low kilovoltage cardiac dual-source CT: attenuation, noise and radiation dose. *Eur Radiol* 2008; 18:1809-1817.

[57] Lau J, Ioannidis JP, Schmid CH. Summing up evidence: one answer is not always enough. *Lancet* 1998; 351: 123-7.

Chapter 11

Coronary CT Angiography in Coronary Artery Disease: How to Use It Wisely and When to Request It Appropriately?

Abstract

Coronary CT angiography has been increasingly used in the diagnosis of coronary artery disease due to rapid technological developments and improved diagnostic performance. High diagnostic accuracy has been achieved with 64- and more slice CT scanners and in selected patients, coronary CT angiography is regarded as a reliable alternative to invasive coronary angiography. Although the tremendous contributions of coronary CT angiography to cardiac imaging are acknowledged, appropriate use of cardiac CT as the first line technique by physicians has not been well established. Optimal selection of cardiac CT is essential to ensure acquisition of valuable diagnostic information and avoid unnecessary invasive procedures.

This is of paramount importance since coronary CT angiography not only involves patient risk assessment, prediction of major adverse cardiac events, but also impacts physician decision- making on patient management. Applications of CT in cardiac imaging include coronary artery calcium scoring for predicting the patient risk of developing major cardiac events, followed by coronary CT angiography which is commonly used to determine the diagnostic and prognostic accuracy in the coronary artery disease. This chapter presents an overview of the applications of CT in cardiac imaging in terms of coronary calcium scoring and coronary CT angiography. Judicious use of both cardiac CT tools will be discussed with regard to their value in different patient risk groups with the aim of identifying the appropriate criteria for choosing a cardiac CT modality. An effective diagnostic pathway is finally recommended to physicians for appropriate selection of cardiac CT in clinical practice.

Keywords: Coronary artery disease, coronary artery calcium, multislice CT, risk, radiation dose

11.1. Introduction

The diagnosis and management of coronary artery disease (CAD) is increasingly dependent on non-invasive imaging modalities. Recent technological advances have led to a considerable increase in image quality for coronary imaging using multislice CT [1-3]. Numerous studies have shown that coronary CT angiography, as a less-invasive alternative to invasive coronary angiography, has a high diagnostic accuracy for the detection of significant coronary stenosis (≥50% lumen stenosis) when compared to invasive coronary angiography [3-9]. High quality multislice CT (64-slice and beyond) is not only able to provide reliable information on coronary luminal changes, but also has the potential to visualize coronary artery wall morphology, characterize atherosclerotic plaques and identify non-stenotic plaques that may be undetected by invasive coronary angiography. Studies have shown that coronary CT angiography demonstrates high prognostic value in CAD, as it is able to differentiate low-risk from high-risk patients [10-12], with very low rate of adverse cardiac events occurring in patients with normal coronary CT angiography, and significantly high rate of these events in patients with obstructive CAD.

It has been a regular procedure to perform coronary artery calcium (CAC) scoring and coronary CT angiography for the diagnosis of patients with suspected CAD. Results dealing with the incremental prognostic value of CAC scoring used in combination with coronary CT angiography have recently been published [13]. Although satisfactory results have been achieved in these studies, with strengths and weaknesses being addressed, very few studies have specifically examined the clinical applications of coronary CT angiography in the particular target population, or risk stratification and assessment with regard to the judicious use of coronary CT angiography [14-16]. Identification of the exact role of coronary CT angiography in patients from different risk groups is clinically significant as this could lead to unnecessary examinations due to the fact that multislice CT is an imaging modality with high radiation dose. In addition, appropriate selection of coronary CT angiography is of paramount importance for physicians to choose it as a gatekeeper for further diagnostic testing. This chapter explores how physicians should use coronary CT angiography wisely in terms of the clinical value of coronary calcium scoring to predict the extent of coronary artery disease or cardiac events, and coronary CT angiography in patients from different risk groups with a focus on low to intermediate risk patients. The potential value and benefits of coronary CT angiography in asymptomatic patients are also explored. Finally, this chapter looks at when physicians should request coronary CT angiography appropriately from a clinical point of view by following the appropriate imaging pathways.

11.2. Current Status of Coronary CT Angiography in Coronary Artery Disease

With recent progress in the technical developments of multislice CT scanners, images can be acquired in a very short time with high spatial resolution. In particular, the development of 64- or more slice CT scanners allows acquisition of cardiac images with a temporal resolution that is a fraction of the length of the cardiac cycle with an isotropic volume resolution of less than 0.5 mm [9, 17]. Non-diagnostic coronary CT angiography studies have decreased from

15-25% with the early generation of 4- and 16-slice CT scanners to less than 10% with 64-slice CT scanners [17, 18]. The cost of performing a coronary CT angiography examination is much lower than that of an invasive coronary angiography, and is equivalent to an imaging stress test. Unlike invasive coronary angiography, which is associated with procedure-related complications, coronary CT angiography is a less invasive modality with very rare occurrence of complications resulting from CT examinations. Consequently, there has been an extensive interest in the clinical application of coronary CT angiography in the evaluation of patients with suspected CAD.

Most studies have reported the diagnostic accuracy of coronary CT angiography on coronary segment-based, coronary artery vessel-based and patient-based assessment. Several meta-analyses of studies on the use of 64-slice CT reported mean sensitivities and specificities ranging from 85% to 99%, and 86% to 96%, respectively [3, 8, 19, 20]. Given the dependence of positive predictive value and negative predictive value on the prevalence of disease, the relatively high prevalence of significant CAD as determined by invasive coronary angiography in many of these selected study populations compared to the general population raises a concern in appraising the value of coronary CT angiography in clinical practice. It has been shown that significant statistical heterogeneity exists among published studies, with smaller studies reporting higher diagnostic accuracy of coronary CT angiography in CAD [21].

Two recent multicentre studies discussed several methodological limitations of coronary CT angiography, as patients with high calcium scores were excluded from the analysis of one study, while in another study, no segments were excluded from the analysis despite high calcium scores [4, 6]. Therefore, reports of the diagnostic value of coronary CT angiography in CAD in the literature need to be interpreted with caution.

11.3. Coronary Artery Calcium Scoring – Predictive Value

Quantifying the amount of coronary artery calcium with unenhanced CT calcium scoring has been widely accepted as a reliable non-invasive technique for screening risk of future cardiac events [22 23], and is usually quantified by using the Agatston score or scores such as the volume score or calcium mass [24-26].

Clinical application of CAC has been supported by evidence showing that absence of calcium reliably excludes obstructive coronary artery stenoses [27], and that the amount of CAC is a strong predictor for risk assessment of myocardial infarction and sudden cardiac death, independent of conventional coronary risk factors [28-30]. However, the prognostic value of CAC depends on the risk groups as to whether patient risk is reclassified and patient management can be changed based on CAC scores when compared to traditional risk assessments [31].

The Framingham risk score is one of the most commonly used risk-estimation systems, which enables clinicians to estimate cardiovascular risk in asymptomatic patients. It is calculated using traditional risk predictors, including age, gender, total cholesterol, high-density lipoprotein cholesterol, smoking status, and systolic blood pressure, and is represented as a 10-year risk score for the prediction of coronary heart disease events [32].

However, there is growing evidence to show that these traditional risk assessment methods, based on risk factor analysis, have significant limitations when used to guide individual patient therapy [32-24]. CAC score by multislice CT has been increasingly used as an additional assessment tool to evaluate the risk of developing major cardiac events in asymptomatic and symptomatic patients.

11.3.1. Coronary Artery Calcium Scoring–Predictive Value in Asymptomatic Patients

In asymptomatic individuals, zero CAC is associated with a very low (<1% per year) risk of major cardiac events over the next 3-5 years, whereas in asymptomatic patients with extensive coronary calcification, the major cardiac events have been reported to be increased by up to 11-fold [35-37]. Several large population-based studies have reported that in asymptomatic patients without known CAD, CAC is predictive of future cardiac events above and beyond traditional risk factors [38-40]. The recent population-based multi-ethnic study of atherosclerosis, conducted in 6,722 asymptomatic patients belonging to four racial ethnic groups and followed for 3.8 years, showed a significant difference in the prevalence of CAC among different ethnic groups.

Nonetheless, CAC has demonstrated incremental prognostic value over traditional risk factors, with a seven-fold increase in the incidence of cardiac events for Agatston scores >100 when compared with patients with zero CAC [38].

Other studies evaluating the prognostic value of the measurement of CAC have shown that coronary calcification is predictive of cardiac events in asymptomatic patients with different age groups [39-41]. LaMonte *et al* in their study consisting of nearly 11,000 patients ranging from 22 to 96 years of age who underwent a screening medical examination, reported increased cardiac events in patients with coronary calcium scores of 400 or more during a mean follow-up of 3.5 years [40].

In the Prospective Army Coronary Calcium Project among men and women 40 to 45 years of age, Talyor *et al* concluded that the presence of coronary calcium was associated with an increase in the risk of coronary events by a factor of 12 during 3 years of follow-up [39]. Similarly, higher calcium scores were found to be associated with the relative risks of coronary events in the population-based Rotterdam Study of elderly asymptomatic patients [41].

11.3.2. Coronary Artery Calcium Scoring– Prognostic Value in Symptomatic Patients

Coronary calcification is considered only marginally related to the degree of coronary stenosis and it is well known that both obstructive and non-obstructive CAD can occur in the absence of calcification [42-44].

Significantly, coronary stenoses are frequently found to be non-calcified (Figure 11.1), and highly calcified plaques are frequently non-obstructive. Thus, the value of a zero or low calcium score (a low coronary calcium score is defined as an Agatston score of 1 to 100 because a coronary calcium score of 100 is often used as a cut-off point for risk assessment) in symptomatic patients remains unclear. Several studies have reported the presence of obstructive non-calcified plaque in up to 8.7% of symptomatic patients with zero or low calcium score [45-47].

The question has been raised as to whether only using CAC score is a reliable tool to determine the extent of CAD, since non-calcified coronary artery plaque may not be detected. Cheng *et al* reported that low but detectable CAC scores are less reliable in predicting plaque burden due to their association with high overall non-calcified coronary artery plaque [45]. They concluded that low CAC scores are significantly less predictive of prevalence or severity of underlying non-calcified coronary plaque.

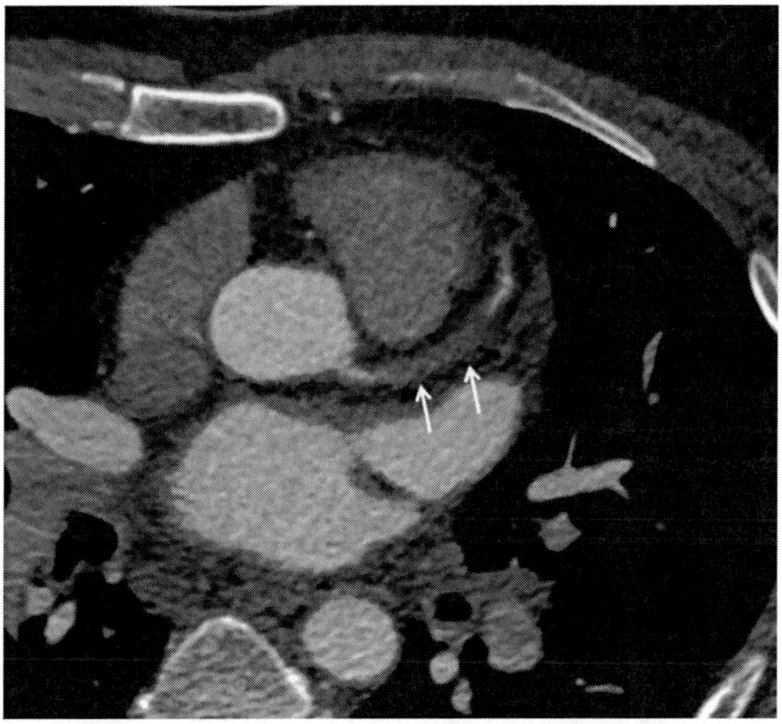

Figure 11.1. Coronary CT angiography in a 43-year-old male presenting with chest pain and raised cardiac enzymes shows non-calcified plaque at the left main and left anterior descending arteries (arrows) causing a complete total occlusion of these vessels.

It has been recently suggested in some studies that coronary CT calcium score assessed with unenhanced CT may be supported by coronary CT angiography, or coronary CT angiography may be performed alone with the aim of acquiring more diagnostic information [48-50]. Coronary CT angiography allows not only visualization of the vessel lumen, but also of the vessel wall, including composition of atherosclerotic plaque (calcified versus non-calcified or mixed type of plaques).

However, the contrast enhancement in the coronary artery vessels may obscure detection of plaque, especially the presence of extensively calcified plaques, and thus may obviate reliable measurements of plaque density. Coronary CT angiography was found to underestimate higher Agatston scores [48]. It has been reported in that study that coronary CT angiography allows for the detection of CAC with high accuracy, as well as good correlation with unenhanced CT calcium score. In contrast, in patients with zero or low calcium score, coronary CT angiography was found to provide additional valuable information on patient management as coronary CT angiography detected obstructive coronary lesions in 7% of patients with a zero score and in 17% with a low CAC score.

Their study indicated that in symptomatic patients with a zero or low CAC score on CT CAC scoring can be used to exclude an acute or long-term coronary syndrome, whereas coronary CT angiography is recommended as the non-invasive test of choice in these patients [48]. Similarly, van Werkhoven *et al* in their recent report showed that coronary CT angiography provided additional prognostic information regarding stenosis severity and plaque composition when compared to CAC score for risk stratification in patients with suspected CAD.

Their study involved analysis of plaque composition with coronary CT angiography, and results showed that the number of segments with non-calcified plaques and the number of segments with mixed plaques was found to be independently associated with increased risk for adverse cardiac events [50].

11.4. Coronary CT Angiography in High-Risk Patients

The pre-test probability of CAD may have a significant impact on the diagnostic performance of the CT scan. Pre-test probability or likelihood is defined according to Diamond and Ferrester criteria, which are based on age, gender and symptomatic status [51]. Intermediate likelihood is defined as a pre-test probability between 13.4% and 87.2%, while low and high pre-test probability are defined as less than 13.4% and more than 87.2%, respectively. It is noticed that the diagnostic performance of coronary CT angiography is different in patients from different risk groups.

The diagnostic accuracy of coronary CT angiography has been extensively studied in populations with a high pre-test likelihood for CAD [17-20]. However, this population is unlikely to benefit from coronary CT angiography because most patients require invasive coronary angiography for the purpose of revascularization. Meijboom *et al* in their prospective study observed that, in patients with a high pre-test likelihood for CAD, interpretations using coronary CT angiography failed to significantly change the post-test probability of significant CAD.

Thus, normal findings of coronary CT angiography did not result in a sufficient reduction of the post-test probability to reliably rule out the presence of significant CAD. These data indicate that the majority of these symptomatic patients are likely to proceed to invasive coronary angiography despite the negative coronary CT angiography findings [15]. Coronary CT angiography is considered to be of limited clinical value in the evaluation of the high pre-test probability group.

In patients with a high pre-test likelihood for significant stenosis, functional evaluation, such as myocardial perfusion imaging, may be more relevant than coronary CT angiography to determine the need for revascularization.

11.5. Coronary CT Angiography in Low- And Intermediate- Risk Patients

In contrast to the high pre-test probability group, patients with an intermediate or low pre-test likelihood for CAD might receive more benefit from coronary CT angiography. A very high negative predictive value (>99%) of coronary CT angiography reliably rules out the presence of significant CAD and can be used as a highly effective gatekeeper for invasive coronary angiography [14, 52, 53]. Thus, when coronary CT angiography is used in a patient population with a low or intermediate pre-test likelihood, the need for additional imaging will be restricted to those patients with an abnormal finding from coronary CT angiography. Consequently, the use of coronary CT angiography could avoid invasive coronary angiography in most patients. This concept is also supported by relevant data about cost-effectiveness. Min *et al* investigated the value of coronary CT angiography as a first line test compared to myocardial perfusion imaging using single photon emission computed tomography (SPECT) in patients with a low to intermediate pre-test likelihood. They concluded that lower referral rates to invasive coronary angiography and lower healthcare costs were observed in their low-risk group [54].

Diagnostic value of coronary CT angiography in the detection of atherosclerosis in low- to intermediate-risk groups has been confirmed in a latest study performed by 64-slice CT compared to myocardial perfusion imaging. Iwasaki *et al* in their study used 64-slice CT to detect subclinical atherosclerosis in 415 asymptomatic patients with more than 95% belonging to low- and intermediate-risk groups [55]. Their results showed very high prevalence (71%) of subclinical atherosclerosis in patients with low to intermediate risk patients, with one-fifth of them having significant coronary stenosis. This is supported by other studies showing the high prevalence of atherosclerosis. Hausleiter *et al* reported the prevalence of coronary plaques was 67.1% in their study comprising of 161 patients with an intermediate risk for coronary artery disease [46]. Choi *et al* studied 1000 middle-aged asymptomatic patients with 64-slice CT and noticed the prevalence of 22% atherosclerotic plaques in these patients [56]. These studies further testified that coronary CT angiography is a valuable imaging modality for detection of atherosclerotic changes in the low- to intermediate-risk patients.

11.6. Coronary CT Angiography in Asymptomatic Patients

Despite the high diagnostic accuracy of coronary artery stenosis and prognostic power of coronary CT angiography in symptomatic patients, to date there have been very limited publications evaluating the prognostic potential of coronary CT angiography in asymptomatic patients. Although only limited data are available in asymptomatic patient populations, it is possible that coronary CT angiography is valuable for risk stratification in these patients, since coronary CT angiography can be used to detect atherosclerosis for long-term risk assessment [57-59]. The prevalence of atherosclerosis was reported to be 22% in a recent study consisting of 1,000 asymptomatic individuals undergoing coronary CT angiography, with 5% and 2% being observed in ≥50% CAD and ≥75% CAD, respectively [57]. Cardiac events occurred in 1.5% of individuals during a follow-up of 17 months, all of whom had atherosclerosis on coronary CT angiography. These data indicate that coronary CT angiography is currently not acceptable as a general screening tool and CAC score testing may be a preferable option. However, non-invasive coronary CT angiography may potentially be used as a test in the workup of asymptomatic individuals with cardiac risk characteristics [57-60].

It has been recently confirmed that performing coronary CT angiography before invasive coronary angiography is a cost-effective strategy in the management of patients without symptoms who have positive stress rest results [59]. It is generally believed that a patient at low risk who has a positive stress test result (such as treadmill ECG studies, stress echocardiography, and radionuclide stress studies) is often referred for cardiac catheterization, especially when the positive stress test result is obtained in a preoperative workup. Halpern *et al* in their study using decision tree analysis reported that when a patient with an expected CAD prevalence of less than 85% is found to have a positive test result, coronary CT angiography is a less expensive alternative to invasive coronary angiography [59]. Although most patients undergo screening for CAD with stress tests to obtain functional and perfusion information which is not available with coronary CT angiography, a meta-analysis on more than 35,000 patients with coronary angiography as the reference standard showed that only average sensitivity and specificity was achieved with stress echocardiography and SPECT [61]. Thus, the use of coronary CT angiography in asymptomatic patients can avoid unnecessary invasive cardiac angiography procedures.

Summary and Conclusion

The introduction of coronary CT angiography has significantly changed the clinical diagnostic approach to CAD. There is no doubt that, in patients with clinical suspected CAD, coronary CT angiography plays a significant role in establishing or excluding the diagnosis. With a very high negative predictive value, coronary CT angiography is widely regarded as a reliable technique in clinical practice to exclude significant CAD.

Use of coronary CT angiography for diagnosis and risk assessment in patients with low or intermediate risk or pretest probability for coronary artery disease is favourably preferred, whereas in high-risk patients, coronary CT angiography is less favourably recommended. Use of non-contrast CT for coronary artery calcium scoring is considered an appropriate approach in low- and intermediate-risk patients for prediction of cardiac events, while in symptomatic or high- risk patients, its predictive value is less reliable due to high prevalence of non-calcified plaques. Appropriate selections of cardiac CT will have a significant impact on physician decision-making and performance that will guide appropriate patient management strategies. Figure 11.2 is a flow chart that recommends the CT imaging pathways for physicians to choose coronary CT angiography appropriately in patients with suspected coronary artery disease and within different pre-test probabilities or risk groups. It is expected that these imaging pathways will assist physicians, particularly cardiologists, to make judicious use of cardiac CT in their clinical practice.

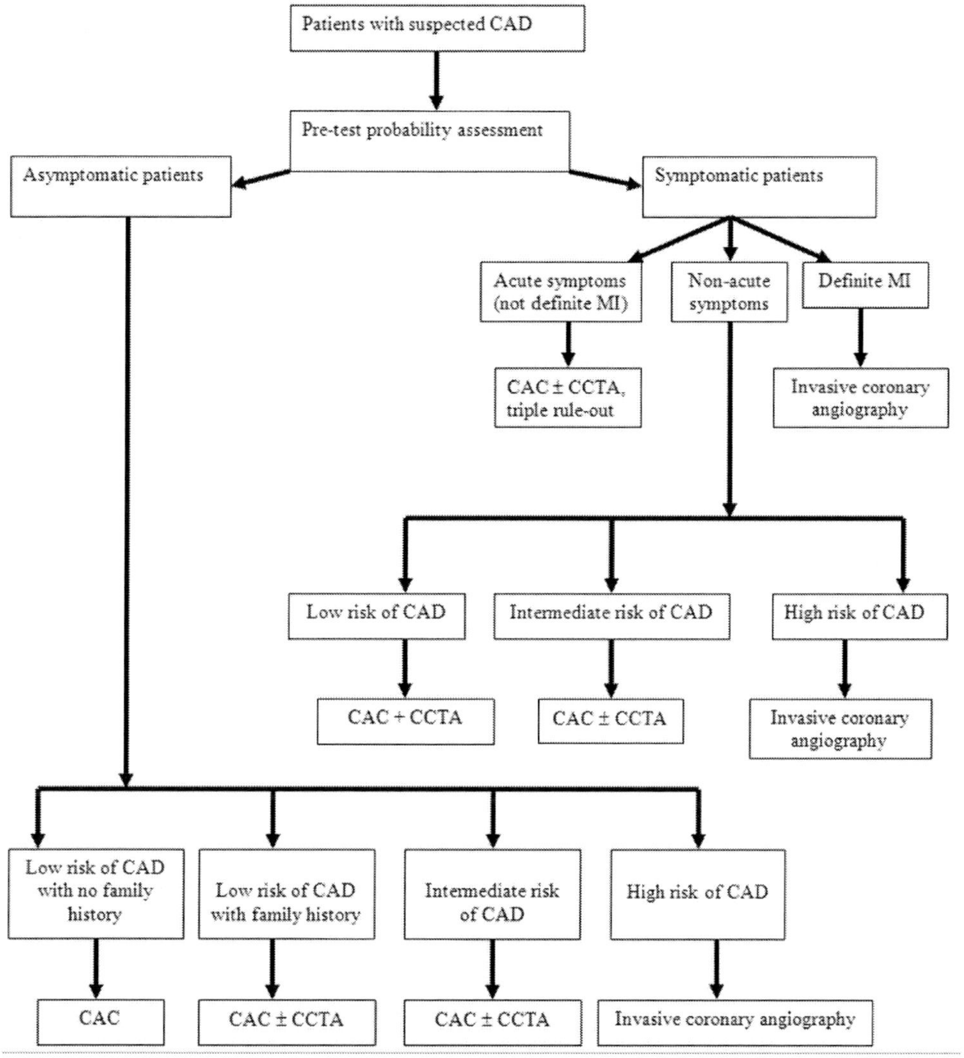

Figure 11.2. Flow chart shows the imaging pathways for appropriate selection of coronary CT angiography in patients with suspected CAD. CAD-coronary artery disease, CCTA-coronary CT angiography, CAC-coronary artery calcium, MI-myocardial infarction.

References

[1] Raff GL, Gallagher MJ, O'Neill WW, Goldstein JA. Diagnostic accuracy of non-invasive coronary angiography using 64-slice spiral computed tomography. *J Am Coll Cardiol* 2005, 46: 552-557.

[2] Wintersperger BJ, Nikolaou K, von Ziegler F, et al. Image quality, motion artifacts, and reconstruction timing of 64-slice coronary computed tomography angiography with 0.33-second rotation speed. *Invest Radiol* 2006;41: 436–442.

[3] Sun Z, Lin CH, Davidson R, et al. Diagnostic value of 64-slice CT angiography in coronary artery disease: A systematic review. *Eur J Radiol* 2008; 67: 78-84.

[4] Miller JM, Rochitte CE, Dewey M, et al. Diagnostic performance of coronary angiography by 64-row CT. *N Engl J Med* 2008; 359: 2324-2326.

[5] Schuijf JD, Pundziute G, Jukema JW, et al. Diagnostic accuracy of 64-slice multislice computed tomography in the noninvasive evaluation of significant coronary artery disease. *Am J Cardiol* 2006;98:145–148.

[6] Budoff MJ, Dowe D, Jollis JG, et al. Diagnostic performance of 64-multidetector row coronary computed tomographic angiography for evaluation of coronary artery stenosis in individuals without known coronary artery disease: results from the prospective multicenter ACCURACY (Assessment by Coronary Computed Tomographic Angiography of Individuals Undergoing Invasive Coronary Angiography) trial. *J Am Coll Cardiol* 2008;52:1724-1732.

[7] Meijboom WB, Meijs MFL, Schuijf JD, et al. Diagnostic accuracy of 64-slice computed tomography coronary angiography: a prospective multicenter, multivendor study. *J Am Coll Cardiol* 2008;52:2135-2144.

[8] Abdulla J, Abildstrom SZ, Gotzsche O, et al. 64-Multislice detector computed tomography coronary angiography as potential alternative to conventional coronary angiography: a systematic review and meta-analysis. *Eur Heart J* 2007;28:3042–3050.

[9] Sun Z, GH Choo, Ng KH. Coronary CT angiography: current status and continuing challenges. *Br J Radiol* 2012; 85: 495-510.

[10] Carrigan TP, Nair D, Schoenhagen P, et al. Prognostic utility of 64-slice computed tomography in patients with suspected but no documented coronary artery disease. *Eur Heart J* 2009; 30:362-371.

[11] Min JK, Feignouz J, Treutenaere J, et al. The prognostic value of multidetector coronary CT angiography for the prediction of major adverse cardiac events: a major multicenter observational cohort study. *Int J Cardiovasc Imaging* 2010; 26: 721-728.

[12] Abdulla J, Asferg C, Kofoed KF. Prognostic value of absence or presence of coronary artery disease determined by 64-slice computed tomography coronary angiography: a systematic review and meta-analysis. *Int J Cardiovasc Imaging* 2011; 27: 413-420.

[13] Ostrom MP, Gopal A, Ahmadi N, et al. Mortality incidence and the severity of coronary atherosclerosis assessed by computed tomography angiography. *J Am Coll Cardiol* 2008; 52: 1335-1343.

[14] van Werkhoven JM, Gaemperli O, Schuijf JD, et al. Multislice computed tomography coronary angiography for risk stratification in patients with an intermediate pretest likelihood. *Heart* 2009; 95: 1607-1611.

[15] Meijboom WB, Van Mieghem CA, Mollet NR, et al. 64-slice computed tomography coronary angiography in patients with high, intermediate, or low pretest probability of significant coronary artery disease. *J Am Coll Cardiol* 2007;50:1469–1475.

[16] Henneman MM, Schuijf JD, van Werkhoven JM, et al. Multi-slice computed tomography coronary angiography for ruling out suspected coronary artery disease: what is the prevalence of a normal study in a general clinical population? *Eur Heart J* 2008;29:2006–2013.

[17] Nasis A, Leung MC, Antonis PR, et al. Diagnostic accuracy of non-invasive coronary angiography with 320-detector row computed tomography. *Am J Cardiol* 2010; 106: 1429-1435.

[18] Sun Z, Jiang W. Diagnostic value of multislice CT angiography in coronary artery disease: A meta-analysis. *Eur J Radiol* 2006; 60: 279-286.

[19] Vanhoenacker PK, Heijenbrok-Kal MH, Van Heste R, Decramer I, Van Hoe LR, Wijns W, et al. Diagnostic performance of multidetector CT angiography for assessment of coronary artery disease: meta-analysis. *Radiology* 2007; 244: 419-428.

[20] Mowatt G, Cook JA, Hillis GS, et al. 64-slice computed tomography angiography in the diagnosis and assessment of coronary artery disease: systematic review and meta-analysis. *Heart* 2008; 94: 1386–1393.

[21] Hamon M, Biondi-Zoccai GG, Malagutti P, et al. Diagnostic performance of multislice spiral computed tomography of coronary arteries as compared with conventional invasive coronary angiography: a meta-analysis. *J Am Coll Cardiol* 2006; 48:1896-1910.

[22] Oudkerk M, Stillman AE, Halliburton SS, et al. Coronary artery calcium screening: current status and recommendations from the European Society of Cardiac Radiology and North American Society for Cardiovascular Imaging. *Int J Cardiovasc Imaging* 2008; 24:645–671.

[23] Greenland P, Bonow RO, Brundage BH, et al. ACCF/AHA 2007 clinical expert consensus document on coronary artery calcium scoring by computed tomography in global cardiovascular risk assessment and in evaluation of patients with chest pain: a report of the American College of Cardiology Foundation Clinical Expert Consensus Task Force (ACCF/AHA Writing Committee to Update the 2000 Expert Consensus Document on Electron Beam Computed Tomography). *Circulation* 2007; 115:402–426.

[24] Agatston AS, Janowitz WR, Hildner FJ, et al. Quantification of coronary artery calcium using ultrafast computed tomography. *J Am Coll Cardiol* 1990; 15:827–832.

[25] Callister TQ, Cooil B, Raya SP, et al. Coronary artery disease: improved reproducibility of calcium scoring with an electron-beam CT volumetric method. *Radiology* 1998; 208:807–814.

[26] Hoffmann U, Siebert U, Bull-Stewart A, et al. Evidence for lower variability of coronary artery calcium mineral mass measurements by multidetector computed tomography in a community based cohort—consequences for progression studies. *Eur J Radiol* 2006; 57:396–402.

[27] Haberl R, Becker A, Leber A, et al. Correlation of coronary calcification and angiographically documented stenoses in patients with suspected coronary artery disease: results of 1,764 patients. *J Am Coll Cardiol* 2001;37:451– 457.

[28] Keelan PC, Bielak LF, Ashai K, et al. Long-term prognostic value of coronary calcification detected by electron-beam computed tomography in patients undergoing coronary angiography. *Circulation* 2001; 104:412–417.

[29] Wong ND, Hsu JC, Detrano RC, et al. Coronary artery calcium evaluation by electron beam computed tomography and its relation to new cardiovascular events. *Am J Cardiol* 2000; 86:495–498.

[30] Arad Y, Spadaro LA, Goodman K, et al. Prediction of coronary events with electron beam computed tomography. *J Am Coll Cardiol* 2000; 36:1253–1260.

[31] National Cholesterol Education Program (NCEP) Expert Panel on Detection. Evaluation, and Treatment of High Blood Cholesterol in Adults (Adult Treatment Panel III). Third report of the National Cholesterol Education Program (NCEP) Expert Panel on Detection, Evaluation, and Treatment of High Blood Cholesterol in Adults (Adult Treatment Panel III) final report. *Circulation* 2002;106:3143-3142

[32] Johnson KM, Dowe DA, Brink JA. Traditional clinical risk assessment tools do not accurately predict coronary atherosclerotic plaque burden: a CT angiography study. *AJR Am J Roentgenol* 2009;192:235-243.
[33] Akosah KO, Schaper A, Cogbill C, et al. Preventing myocardial infarction in the young adult in the first place: how do the National Cholesterol Education Panel III guidelines perform? *J Am Coll Cardiol* 2003;41:1475-1479.
[34] Nasir K, Michos ED, Blumenthal RS, et al. Detection of high-risk young adults and women by coronary calcium and National Cholesterol Education Program Panel III guidelines. *J Am Coll Cardiol* 2005;46: 1931-1936.
[35] Greenland P, Bonow RO, Brundage BH, et al. ACCF/AHA 2007 clinical expert consensus document on coronary artery calcium scoring by computed tomography in global cardiovascular risk assessment and in evaluation of patients with chest pain: a report of the American College of Cardiology Foundation Clinical Expert Consensus Task Force (ACCF/ AHA Writing Committee to Update the 2000 Expert Consensus Document on Electron Beam Computed Tomography) developed in collaboration with the Society of Atherosclerosis Imaging and Prevention and the Society of Cardiovascular Computed Tomography. *J Am Coll Cardiol* 2007;49:378–402.
[36] Detrano R, Guerci AD, Carr JJ, et al. Coronary calcium as a predictor of coronary events in four racial or ethnic groups. *N Engl J Med* 2008;358:1336–1345.
[37] Sarwar A, Shaw LJ, Shapiro MD, et al. Diagnostic and prognostic value of absence of coronary artery calcification. *JACC Cardiovasc Imaging* 2009;2: 675–688.
[38] Budoff MJ, Nasir K, McClelland RL, et al. Coronary calcium predicts events better with absolute calcium scores than age-sex-race/ethnicity percentiles: MESA (Multi-Ethnic Study of Atherosclerosis). *J Am Coll Cardiol* 2009;53:345–352.
[39] Taylor AJ, Bindeman J, Feuerstein I, et al. Coronary calcium independently predicts incident premature coronary heart disease over measured cardiovascular risk factors: mean three-year outcomes in the Prospective Army Coronary Calcium (PACC) project. *J Am Coll Cardiol* 2005;46:807–814.
[40] LaMonte MJ, FitzGerald SJ, Church TS, et al. Coronary artery calcium score and coronary heart disease events in a large cohort of asymptomatic men and women. *Am J Epidemiol* 2005;162:421-429.
[41] Vliegenthart R, Oudkerk M, Hofman A, et al. Coronary calcification improves cardiovascular risk prediction in the elderly. *Circulation* 2005;112:572-577.
[42] Gottlieb I, Miller JM, Arbab-Zadeh A, et al.: The absence of coronary calcification does not exclude obstructive coronary artery disease or the need for revascularization in patients referred for conventional coronary angiography. *J Am Coll Cardiol* 2010, 55:627–634.
[43] Chang SM, Nabi F, Xu J, et al. The coronary artery calcium score and stress myocardial perfusion imaging provide independent and complementary prediction of cardiac risk. *J Am Coll Cardiol* 2009, 54:1872–1882.
[44] Lau GT, Ridley LJ, Schieb MC, et al. Coronary artery stenoses: detection with calcium scoring, CT angiography, and both methods combined. *Radiology* 2005, 235:415–422.
[45] Cheng VY, Lepor NE, Madyoon H, et al. Presence and severity of noncalcified coronary plaque on 64-slice computed tomographic coronary angiography in patients with zero and low coronary artery calcium. *Am J Cardiol* 2007; 99:1183–1186.

[46] Hausleiter J, Meyer T, Hadamitzky M, et al. Prevalence of noncalcified coronary plaques by 64-slice computed tomography in patients with an intermediate risk for significant coronary artery disease. *J Am Coll Cardiol* 2006; 48: 312-318.

[47] Akram K, O'Donnell RE, King S, et al. Influence of symptomatic status on the prevalence of obstructive coronary artery disease in patients with zero calcium score. *Atherosclerosis* 2009; 203: 533-537.

[48] Rubinshtein R, Gaspar T, Halon DA, et al. Prevalence and extent of obstructive coronary artery disease in patients with zero or low calcium score undergoing 64-slice cardiac multidetector computed tomography for evaluation of a chest pain syndrome. *Am J Cardiol* 2007; 99:472–475.

[49] van der Bijl N, Joemai RMS, Geleijns J, et al. Assessment of Agatston coronary artery calcium score using contrast-enhanced CT coronary angiography. *AJR Am J Roentgenol* 2010; 195: 1299-1305.

[50] van Werkhoven, Shuijf JD, Gaemperli O, et al. Incremental prognostic value of multi-slice computed tomography coronary angiography over coronary artery calcium scoring in patients with suspected coronary artery disease. *Eur Heart J* 2009; 30: 2622-2629.

[51] Diamond GA, Forrester JS. Analysis of probability as an aid in the clinical diagnosis of coronary-artery disease. *N Engl J Med* 1979;300:1350–1358.

[52] Leber AW, Johnson T, Becker A, et al. Diagnostic accuracy of dual-source multi-slice CT-coronary angiography in patients with an intermediate pretest likelihood for coronary artery disease. *Eur Heart J* 2007;28:2354 –2360.

[53] van Werkhoven JM, Heijenbrok MW, Schuijf JD, et al. Diagnostic accuracy of 64-slice multislice computed tomographic coronary angiography in patients with an intermediate pretest likelihood for coronary artery disease. *Am J Cardiol* 2010; 105: 302-305.

[54] Min JK, Kang N, Shaw LJ, et al. Costs and clinical outcomes after coronary multidetector CT angiography in patients without known coronary artery disease: comparison to myocardial perfusion SPECT. *Radiology* 2008;249:62–70.

[55] Iwasaki K, Matsumoto T, Aono H, et al. Prevalence of subclinical atherosclerosis in asymptomatic patients with low-to-intermediate risk by 64-slice computed tomography. *Coron Artery Dis* 2010; 22: 18-25.

[56] Choi EK, Choi SI, Rivera JJ, et al. Coronary computed tomography angiography as a screening tool for the detection of occult coronary artery disease in asymptomatic individuals. *J Am Coll Cardiol* 2008;52:357-365.

[57] Hadamitzky M, Meyer T, Hein F, et al. Prognostic value of coronary computed tomographic angiography in asymptomatic patients. *Am J Cardiol* 2010; 105: 1746 – 1751.

[58] van Werkhoven JM, Bax JJ, Nucifora G, et al. The value of multi-slice-computed tomography coronary angiograhy for risk stratification. *J Nucl Cardiol* 2009; 16: 970-980.

[59] Halpern EJ, Savage MP, Fischman DL, Levin DC. Cost-effectiveness of coronary CT angiography in evaluation of patients without symptoms who have positive stress test results. *AJR Am J Roentgenol* 2010; 194: 1257-1262.

[60] Hwang Y, Kim Y, Chung IM, et al. Coronary heart disease risk assessment and characterization of coronary artery disease using coronary CT angiography: comparison of asymptomatic and symptomatic groups. *Clin Radiol* 2010; 65: 601-608.

[61] Heijenbrok-Kal MH, Fleischmann KE, Hunink MG. Stress echocardiography, stress single-photon-emission computed tomography and electron beam computed tomography for the assessment of coronary artery disease: a meta-analysis of diagnostic performance. *Am Heart J* 2007; 154:415–423

Chapter 12

Coronary CT Angiography: Current Status and Continuing Challenges

Abstract

Coronary CT angiography represents one of the most exciting advances in the medical imaging field and it has been increasingly used in the diagnosis of coronary artery disease due to rapid technological developments. Although satisfactory results have been reported in the literature with use of 64- and more slice CT, there exist a number of challenges and controversies with respect to the diagnostic accuracy and appropriate use of coronary CT angiography in patients with suspected coronary artery disease. The purpose of this chapter is to discuss the diagnostic role of coronary CT angiography in the workup of coronary artery disease, including technical and diagnostic challenges; diagnostic value of coronary CT angiography in patients from different risk groups; radiation dose issue; awareness of radiation dose by physicians and patients; and finally when physicians should refer coronary CT angiography to patients with suspected coronary artery disease.

Keywords: Coronary artery disease, coronary CT angiography, radiation dose, risk

12.1. Introduction

Coronary artery disease (CAD) remains the leading cause of death in many advanced countries and its prevalence is increasing among developing countries [1, 2]. In 2001, CAD was reported to be responsible for 7.3 million deaths and 58 million disability-adjusted life years lost worldwide [3]. CAD is the leading cause of cardiovascular death throughout the world. According to recent World Health Organization statistics for 2007, cardiovascular deaths account for 33.7% of all deaths worldwide, whereas cancer represents 29.5%, other chronic diseases 26.5%, injury 7%, and communicable diseases 4.6% [4]. Cardiovascular disease costs more than any other diagnostic group [1]. The total direct and indirect cost of cardiovascular disease and stroke in the United States for 2010 is estimated to be $503.2

billion. In contrast, in 2008, the estimated cost of all cancer and benign neoplasms was $228 billion. In light of the current global focus on healthcare utilization, costs, and quality, it is essential to monitor and understand the magnitude of healthcare delivery and costs, as well as the quality of healthcare delivery in relation to the CAD. Invasive coronary angiography is widely used as a reliable technique to diagnose CAD because of its superior spatial and temporal resolution. However, it is an invasive and expensive procedure with associated morbidity and mortality [5]. Furthermore, invasive coronary angiography usually requires a short hospital stay and causes discomfort for the patients. Therefore, a non-invasive technique for imaging of the coronary artery disease is highly desirable. The diagnosis and management of CAD is increasingly dependent on non-invasive imaging modalities. Over the last decades, non-invasive coronary imaging modalities have undergone rapid developments, such as electron-beam CT (EBCT) and magnetic resonance imaging [6, 7]. Despite encouraging results, neither of these techniques has been considered suitable for routine clinical use in the diagnosis of CAD. Imaging of the heart and coronary artery tree has moved into a new diagnostic era with the introduction of multislice CT and development of electrocardiography-synchronized scanning and reconstruction techniques [8, 9]. Recent technological advances have led to a considerable increase in image quality for coronary imaging using multislice CT. Numerous studies have shown that coronary CT angiography has a high diagnostic accuracy for the detection of significant CAD (>50% lumen stenosis) when compared to invasive coronary angiography [10-13]. High quality multislice CT (64-slice and higher) is not only able to provide reliable information on coronary luminal changes, but also has the potential to visualize morphological changes of the coronary artery wall, characterize atherosclerotic plaques and identify non-stenotic plaques that may be undetected by invasive coronary angiography. Studies have shown that coronary CT angiography demonstrates high prognostic value in CAD, as it is able to differentiate low-risk from high-risk patients [14, 15], with very low rate of adverse cardiac events occurring in patients with normal coronary CT angiography, and significantly high rate of these events in patients with obstructive CAD. Although satisfactory results have been achieved with coronary CT angiography, and in selected patients, it is recommended as a reliable alternative to invasive coronary angiography, there are controversial reports in the literature with regard to the diagnostic value of coronary CT angiography. In addition, a number of challenges exist for coronary CT angiography before it becomes a routine imaging modality to replace invasive coronary angiography. This chapter focuses on exploration of the technical, clinical and diagnostic challenges of coronary CT angiography in the diagnosis of CAD. Controversial areas are also explored, such as variable reports of diagnostic value of coronary CT angiography in the literature due to different study designs; when coronary CT angiography should be referred by physicians to patients for CAD detection and diagnosis, and whether coronary CT angiography is appropriately selected and utilized as a first line technique for reduction of the unnecessary invasive angiography examinations.

12.2. Technical Challenges of Coronary CT Angiography

To acquire images with minimal or no artefacts due to cardiac motion, very short exposure times are required for the acquisition of axial images of the heart and coronary artery. High temporal resolution is particularly important for imaging the coronary artery and its branches as they are located very close to the myocardium and demonstrate strong movement during cardiac cycle. Traditionally, non-invasive imaging of the heart and coronary artery is performed with contrast-enhanced EBCT due to its high temporal resolution (50-100 ms). However, the diagnostic value of sensitivity and specificity of EBCT is limited because of the low spatial resolution (1.5 mm to 3.0 mm along the longitudinal axis). This restricts its diagnostic value in accurately evaluating the severity of coronary artery disease. After the arrival of multislice CT scanners in the late 1990s, the use of EBCT became scarce and was eventually replaced by multislice CT from 2003 onwards.

Improved temporal resolution in cardiac CT is achieved by fast rotation of the X-ray tube, but even more importantly by a dedicated reconstruction algorithm [16]. The temporal resolution of multislice CT scanners is essentially determined by the speed of gantry rotation. The half-scan reconstruction technique is the method of choice in all modern multislice CT scanners for image reconstruction in cardiac CT applications. A temporal resolution of about 250 ms is estimated to be appropriate for motion free imaging in the diastolic phase up to a heart rate of about 60 beats per minute (bpm), about 200 ms up to a heart rate of 70 bpm, and approximately 100-150 ms for imaging heart rates up to 90 or even higher bpm [17, 18]. The temporal resolution for 4-slice CT is 250 ms which restricts the diagnostic applications of coronary CT angiography to a greater extent. With 16- and 64-slice CT, the temporal resolution is reduced to 165 ms, and to 75 ms with dual-source CT (even down to 37.5 ms using 2-segment reconstruction algorithm) [19], thus, diagnostic performance of coronary CT angiography has been improved significantly. Therefore, there is a strong demand for the improvement of temporal resolution of multislice CT scanners, so that coronary CT angiography can be extended to image patients with high heart rates. Improvement of spatial resolution in multislice CT is of particular importance for the evaluation of CT coronary calcification scoring and coronary CT angiography. Many cardiac structures, especially the coronary arteries and corresponding side branches represent small and complex 3D structures that require very high and submillimeter isotropic spatial resolution with longitudinal resolution close or equal to in-plane resolution (0.4-0.6 mm) [17]. With early generation of multislice CT scanners such as 4-slice CT, the diagnostic accuracy is limited due to inferior spatial resolution, and the unassessable segments could be as high as more than 30% in studies performed with 4-slice CT [20]. With the introduction of 16- and 64- slice CT, and the development of 256- and 320-slice CT, acquisition of isotropic volume data is made available (isotropic voxel 0.5 x 0.5 x 0.5 mm^3 or 0.6 x 0.6 x 0.6 mm^3), thus detection of main and side coronary artery branches is significantly improved when compared to earlier types of multislice CT scanners [10, 20]. In summary, isotropic volume data is available with 64- or more slice CT scanners, which enables excellent visualization of both main and side branches of coronary artery tree. The temporal resolution of current multislice CT scanners is still inferior to that of invasive coronary angiography. However, with developments of dual-source CT (DSCT) and use of reconstruction algorithms, it is possible to achieve a temporal resolution between 37.5 ms and 75 ms, thus, imaging patients with high heart rates or no need to control heart rates has become a reality. Table 12.1 lists the technical details of different generations of the multislice CT scanners.

Table 12.1. Technical details in terms of spatial and temporal resolution for different generations of multislice CT scanners

Maximum Resolution	4-slice CT	16-slice CT	64-slice CT		256-slice CT	320-slice CT	Invasive coronary angiography
			Single-source	Dual-source			
Maximum Spatial resolution (x, y, z-axis mm^3)	0.6 x 0.6 x 1.0	0.5 x 0.5 x 0.6	0.5 x 0.5 x 0.5/ 0.6 x 0.6 x0.6	0.5 x 0.5 x 0.5/ 0.6 x 0.6 x0.6	0.67 x 0.67 x 0.67	0.5 x 0.5 x 0.5	0.2 x 0.2
Maximum Temporal resolution (ms)	250	165	165	75	135	175	10

12.3. Diagnostic Challenges of Coronary CT Angiography

Over the last decade a great deal of interest has been focused on imaging and diagnosis of CAD using multislice CT, due to its less invasive nature and improved spatial and temporal resolution. Moderate to high diagnostic accuracy was achieved with 64- or more slice CT, owing to further technical improvements [10, 21-24]. These studies have indicated that coronary CT angiography has high accuracy for the diagnosis of CAD and could be used as an effective alternative to invasive coronary angiography in selected patients. However, there are a number of challenges that need to be resolved with respect to the diagnostic accuracy of coronary CT angiography.

One of the main difficulties for cardiac imaging is that image quality highly depends on heart rate. Despite promising results having been achieved with recent multislice CT scanners, the assessability and diagnostic accuracy are still higher in patients with a lower heart rate, and deteriorate at a higher heart rate [20]. Thus, beta-blockers are frequently used in coronary CT angiography performed with 64- or more slice CT scanners with the aim of lowering the heart rate to less than 65 bpm. DSCT offers improved temporal resolution compared to single-source 64-slice CT, thus, high diagnostic accuracy can still be achieved with use of DSCT in a wide range of patients with higher and even irregular heart rates [25, 26]. Despite slightly lower per-segment evaluablility in patients with higher heart rates, DSCT did not show decrease in diagnostic accuracy for the detection of coronary stenoses [27, 28]. DSCT improves temporal resolution which is vital in those patients who cannot sustain beta blockage or do not respond well to the heart control with use of beta blockers.

It has been well established that the diagnostic value of coronary CT angiography is hindered by the presence of extensive calcification in the coronary artery tree. According to several meta-analyses [20-23], high-density calcification produces blooming artefacts which lead to overestimation of the degree of coronary stenosis, thus resulting in low positive predictive value. Patients with high Agatston calcium scores are generally excluded from studies using coronary CT angiography. Specifically, calcium scores greater than 400 were found to significantly reduce the diagnostic specificity due to high number of false positive cases. This was confirmed by the three recently published prospective studies investigating the effect of high calcium scores or body mass index (BMI) on the diagnostic value of coronary CT angiography [11-13]. Results from these studies showed that a high patient-based specificity of more than 90% was achieved when patients with BMI >40 kg/m^2 and a calcium score of more than 600 were excluded from the analysis, whereas a low to moderate specificity of 64% and 83% was reported in the studies with inclusion of patients with poor image quality and extensive calcification [12, 13]. These conflicting findings indicate the challenge of coronary CT angiography in patients with suspected CAD in the presence of high calcium scores or extensive calcification, or large BMI.

Diagnostic value of coronary CT angiography in CAD is usually assessed according to either patient-based, or vessel-based, or segment-based criterion. However, the reports in the literature should be interpreted with caution as there is a lack of uniform criteria for the assessment of the coronary arteries and associated branches or segments. Studies performed with early generations of multislice CT, such as 4- and 16-slice CT scanners involved assessment of coronary arteries based on a wide variation ranging from 9 to 17-segment classification [20], so this indicates a variation of the data analysis, thus affecting the results to a greater extent. A 15- to 17-segment classification according to American Heart Association is commonly used in the majority of studies performed with 64-slice CT scanners, thus, leading to more consistent results [10, 22-24]. Similarly, a significant variation was reported on a vessel-based evaluation. It is expected that all of the four coronary vessels within any patient should be included in the analysis; however, in some studies, the average coronary arteries per patient to be evaluated ranged from 2.77 to 4.0 [29-31]. In addition, the unevaluable segments (mainly the distal small coronary segments) were excluded from the analysis in most of the studies [10, 20], so this could lead to high diagnostic accuracy in studies performed with 16-slice coronary CT angiography.

Another limitation of coronary CT angiography is the criterion of determining significant coronary stenosis which is set at more than 50% lumen stenosis, as this is normally performed in most of the studies. A recent study has reported that diagnostic performance of coronary CT angiography is optimal for predicting the hemodynamically significant stenosis when the degree of stenosis is more than 60% [32]. Future studies adopting the suitable cut-off value of stenosis degree are required to ensure the validity of diagnostic performance of coronary CT angiography in CAD.

In summary, given the above-mentioned challenges, the reported diagnostic value of coronary CT angiography in the detection and diagnosis of CAD could be variable according to the literature, due to the heterogeneity of study designs. Therefore, standardized protocols should be implemented across institutions with the aim of reducing variation across patients and facilities.

12.4. Radiation Dose Challenges of Coronary CT Angiography

12.4.1. Radiation-Induced Risk and Dose Reduction

Radiation exposure associated with coronary CT angiography has increased substantially over the past two decades and it has raised a major concern in the medical field that needs to draw attention to both clinicians and manufacturers. The general view about radiation dose is that coronary CT angiography is associated with a risk of cancer development [33-36]. Therefore, coronary CT angiography should be performed with dose-saving strategies whenever possible to minimize or reduce the radiation dose to patients.

Effective dose is a single parameter used to reflect the relative risk from exposure to ionizing radiation. The calculation of the effective dose of coronary CT angiography takes into account the biological effect of the radiation on the heart because each organ is given a tissue weighting depending on its individual susceptibility to the effects of ionizing radiation. The tissue weightings are derived from the ICRP (International Commission on Radiological Protection) which focuses on all aspects of protection from ionizing radiation. The conversion factor used to calculate effective dose from coronary CT angiography has been upgraded from 0.014 to 0.028, thus, doses from coronary CT angiography could be significantly underestimated due to failure of using a cardiac specific conversion factor in the recent ICRP documentation [37-39]. Appropriate conversion factors are needed to accurately estimate effective dose. A conversion factor of 0.014 or 0.017 is commonly used in many cardiac CT studies to estimate the effective dose associated with coronary CT angiography, as shown in the previous chapters, thus, this could lead to variable ranges in the reported effective dose. As a result, the dose-length product or CT dose index is recommended to compare the radiation exposure of coronary CT angiography [40].

As the use of cardiac CT continues to grow, particularly in young adult patients, concern over the population dose from CT is being widely expressed in the scientific literature [34, 41, 42]. It has become clear that the responsible use of CT is absolutely necessary in terms of justifying and adjusting scanning techniques. In response to these concerns, the radiology community (radiologists, medical physicists, and manufacturers) has worked to implement ALARA (as low as reasonably achievable) principles in CT imaging [43, 44]. The guiding principle for dose measurement in cardiac CT is that the right dose for a cardiac CT examination takes into account the specific patient attenuation and the specific diagnostic purpose. The reader is referred to several excellent review articles on dose reduction strategies currently recommended in coronary CT angiography [19, 40-43].

For comparison, the radiation dose of diagnostic coronary angiography is between 3 and 9 mSv, while the average yearly background radiation dose is around 2.4 mSv, but this varies between populations [45]. About 10% of people worldwide are exposed to annual effective doses greater than 3 mSv [35]. As shown in the previous chapters, it is possible to produce the radiation dose from coronary CT angiography equivalent to or even lower than that from invasive coronary angiography if appropriate dose-saving strategies are implemented. With most recent multislice CT scanners such as 320-slice CT, whole heart coronary CT angiography has the potential to significantly reduce the radiation dose compared with invasive coronary angiography while maintaining high diagnostic accuracy [46].

12.4.2. Awareness of Radiation Dose

As public awareness of medical radiation exposure has increased recently, there has been intensified awareness among patients, physicians, and regulatory agencies of the importance and need for holistic benefit-and-risk discussions as the basis of information consent in medicine [47]. Communicating benefits and risks of CT scans in a comprehensive manner between physicians and patients is a challenge, as this could lead to potential harm if the patient avoids appropriate and medically necessary imaging because of misunderstanding or unfounded fears [48, 49].

12.4.3. Awareness of Radiation Dose by Physicians

Although ionizing radiation has been established to be linked to the cancer development, with increased concern having been expressed widely in the literature, the knowledge of health care professionals about the radiation doses arising from CT scans is limited and inadequate, regardless of the field of expertise [50-55]. Studies have shown that physicians and radiologists lack awareness of the potential risk associated with common radiological examinations, especially CT imaging [51, 55]. Krille *et al* conducted a systematic review of 14 primary research articles on physicians' knowledge of radiation dose from CT and other diagnostic imaging procedures and associated risks. Their analysis indicated there is a moderate to low level of knowledge and radiation risk awareness among the physicians [55]. Wong *et al* in their recent questionnaire study assessed the general awareness of radiation exposure associated with radiological imaging, and their results indicated that physicians and radiologists' knowledge on radiation dose related to CT imaging is poor and unsatisfactory [56]. This could imply a tendency of radiation misuse and under-utilization of alternative imaging modalities such as ultrasound or magnetic resonance imaging, as some medical practitioners in their survey failed to recognize ultrasound and magnetic resonance imaging as radiation-free modalities. Lee *et al* found that only 47% of radiologists and 9% of emergency department physicians believed that there was an increased risk of cancer associated with CT scans [51]. Jacob *et al* in their questionnaire study reported that only 12.5% of doctors were aware of the 1/2000 risk of induction of a fatal cancer resulting from the abdominal CT scans [52]. Thus, there is an urgent need for physicians to educate themselves and increase their awareness about ionizing radiation from CT and its associated risks.

12.4.4. Awareness of Radiation Dose by Patients

There is a growing trend in medical practice where patients are becoming more involved in medical decision making [57-59]. Prudent and ethical medical practice requires close communication between the patient and the physician. Clearly, shared medical decision making requires a dialogue between patients and their healthcare providers [60]. Degner *et al* found that 44% of patients with breast cancer wanted to make treatment decisions in collaboration with their physician, while 34% wanted to leave the decision to their physician [58]. Similarly, it was reported in a recent study by Caoili *et al* that 83% of their patients stated that they had discussed the reasons for obtaining a CT examination with their physician, and the decision to undergo CT imaging was shared by both the physician and patient in 44% of the cohort [59]. However, the patients' knowledge about ionizing radiation associated with CT examination was limited. Their survey showed that most of the patients were not aware of the risks associated with medical imaging, with only 6% of respondents having knowledge of the information that radiation exposure from CT increased the lifetime risk of cancer.

Some researchers suggested that the referring physician should be the one to explain to patients on radiation-related information [61]. While another approach of increasing awareness of radiation safety could be achieved through providing leaflets and education posters in the hospitals. It has been shown in a study that brief brochures with information about CT scan could improve the understanding of parents of pediatric patients and would not increase refusal rate [62]. In summary, the way we communicate benefit and risk can affect a patient's perceptions and decision making. It is clear that better information and education about medical radiation and the associated benefit and risk consequences are needed, as well as a deeper understanding of the psychology of risk communications [60]. Therefore, increased awareness of radiation dose related to CT scan by both physicians and patients is equally important to ensure the appropriate use and selection of CT imaging technique.

12.5. Controversies-Diagnostic Reports in the Literature

Although promising results have been achieved regarding the diagnostic value of coronary CT angiography in patients with suspected CAD, its role is controversial. As mentioned earlier in the diagnostic challenge, excellent results of coronary CT angiography had been obtained at least in part due to exclusions in some instances of poorly visualized coronary segments or patients with large BMI, high coronary calcium scores, or high heart rates. Other controversial areas include whether coronary artery calcium scoring should be part of the routine coronary CT angiography protocol, and when coronary CT angiography should be referred by physicians to diagnose patients with suspected CAD or to serve for risk stratification purpose.

12.5.1. Should Coronary Calcium Scoring Be Incorporated into Coronary CT Angiography?

There is absolutely no doubt that coronary CT angiography represents the most valuable and potentially effective alternative to invasive coronary angiography for the diagnosis of CAD. Coronary CT angiography has been recommended as an alternative diagnostic modality for evaluating CAD in patients with different risk profiles [63]. Currently, coronary calcium scoring (CAC) has been widely accepted as an effective indicator for screening risk of future cardiac events, independent of traditional risk factors [64-66]. Quantifying the amount of coronary artery calcium with non contrast-enhanced CT calcium scoring is usually performed using the Agatston score. Clinical application of CAC scoring has been supported by evidence showing that absence of calcium reliably excludes obstructive coronary artery stenoses, and that the amount of CAC is a strong predictor for risk assessment of myocardial infarction and sudden cardiac death [67]. However, the role of CAC scoring in patients from different risk groups has been controversial according to the literature and statements from different professional societies. Currently, performing both CAC scoring and coronary CT angiography in combination has been a regular procedure for the diagnosis of CAD. Results dealing with the incremental prognostic value of CAC scoring used in combination with coronary CT angiography have recently been published [68]. Studies have shown that higher CAC scores are associated with increased plaque burden and increased adverse cardiac events [69-71]. Since coronary CT angiography allows not only visualization of the vessel lumen, but also of the vessel wall, including composition of atherosclerotic plaques, several studies have taken advantages of this feature of coronary CT angiography in patients with suspected CAD. Reports from these studies have demonstrated that coronary CT angiography may supplement CAC scoring and could be performed alone to acquire most prognostic information [72-74]. Thus, if CAC scoring has no added benefit over coronary CT angiography in the routinely combined CAC scoring and coronary CT angiography scans, CAC scoring may not be necessarily incorporated into the coronary CT angiography protocol. Kwon *et al* in their recent prospective study concluded that coronary CT angiography has positive correlation with CAC scores for prediction of major adverse cardiac events, and coronary CT angiography has better predictive value than CAC scoring in low-risk patients suspected of CAD [75]. Their results showed no added benefit to the addition of CAC scoring to coronary CT angiography, although their study population was restricted to a relatively low-risk group. Some statements on CAC scoring are available from professional societies, but their views are diverse. In 2000, a consensus statement of the American College of Cardiology and the American Heart Association recommended against CT calcium scoring in asymptomatic individuals [76, 77]. Similarly, statements of the Cardiology Society of Australian and New Zealand and the US Preventive Services Task Force recommend against CT scanning for calcium scoring of coronary stenosis [78, 79]. By comparison, the European guidelines issued on behalf of eight societies are more positive and state that the calcium scoring is an important parameter to detect asymptomatic individuals at high risk for future cardiac events, independent of traditional risk factors [80, 81].

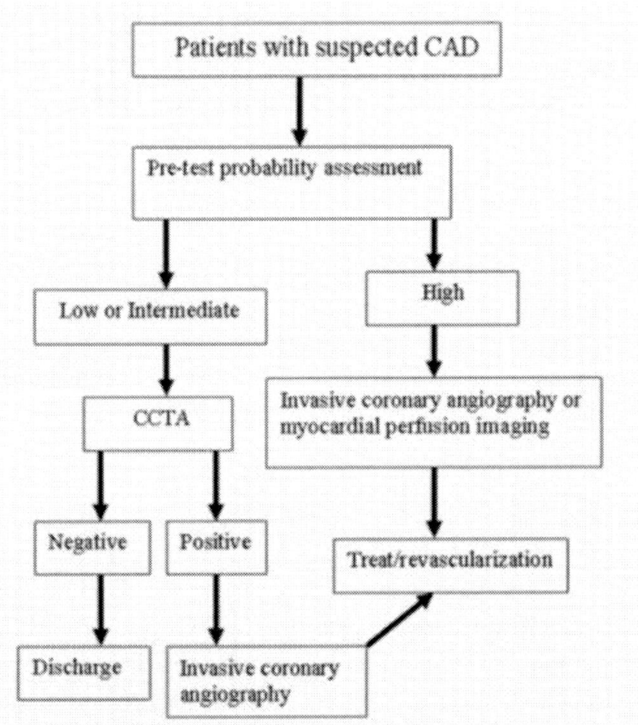

Figure 12.1. Flow chart shows the imaging pathways for appropriate selection of coronary CT angiography in patients with suspected coronary artery disease. CAD-coronary artery disease, CCTA-coronary CT angiography.

Another factor which needs to be considered when using CAC scoring as a screening tool is the radiation dose. CAC scoring is usually performed with a low-radiation dose protocol as the purpose of CT scan is to detect and quantify the calcium rather than diagnosis of CAD. However, it still delivers radiation exposure to patients, although the dose is much lower than that from routine coronary CT angiography. Efstathopoulos *et al* recently reviewed patient radiation dose associated with CAC scoring and coronary CT angiography, and reported that the mean effective dose for CAC scoring with use of retrospective ECG-gating is between 2.7 and 3.3 mSv, while with use of prospective ECG-triggering, the mean dose ranges from 0.7 to 1.1 mSv [82]. Effective dose for coronary CT angiography performed with prospective ECG-triggering ranges from 2.9 to 3.9 mSv. Thus, additional radiation dose from CAC scoring should be taken into account if CAC scoring is recommended as part of the coronary CT angiography protocol.

Figure 11.2 is the flow chart showing recommended imaging pathways with use of CAC scoring and coronary CT angiography in patients with suspected CAD. As shown in the figure, CAC scoring is not recommended in symptomatic patients as coronary calcification is considered only marginally related to the degree of coronary stenosis because both obstructive and non-obstructive CAD can occur in the absence of calcification [83-88]. Low CAC scores are found to be significantly less predictive of prevalence or severity of underlying non-calcified coronary plaque.

12.5.2. When Should Coronary CT Angiography Be Referred by Physicians?

Despite satisfactory results having been reported for coronary CT angiography to diagnose significant coronary artery disease in the literature, it is noticed that the diagnostic performance of coronary CT angiography is different in patients from different risk groups. Thus, judicious use of coronary CT angiography by physicians who request the coronary CT angiography examination has become an important factor in justifying the selection of coronary CT angiography in clinical practice. The diagnostic accuracy of coronary CT angiography has been widely studied in populations with a high pre-test likelihood for CAD (e.g. with typical angina, risk factors and a positive stress test) [20-23, 89]. However, this population should not undergo coronary CT angiography as it is unlikely for them to benefit from coronary CT angiography because most patients would probably be better served by undergoing invasive coronary angiography for the purpose of revascularization. Meijboom *et al* in their prospective study observed that, in patients with a high pre-test probability for CAD, interpretations using coronary CT angiography failed to significantly change the post-test probability of significant CAD [63]. Thus, normal findings of coronary CT angiography did not result in a sufficient reduction of the post-test probability to reliably rule out the presence of significant CAD. These data indicate that the majority of these symptomatic patients are likely to proceed to invasive coronary angiography despite the negative coronary CT angiography findings. In patients with a high pre-test probability for significant stenosis, functional evaluation, such as myocardial perfusion imaging, may be more relevant than coronary CT angiography to determine the need for revascularization [90].

In contrast to the high pre-test probability group, patients with an intermediate or low pre-test likelihood for CAD might receive more benefit from coronary CT angiography. The most obvious indication for coronary CT angiography is to exclude CAD in patients with low to intermediate pretest likelihood of disease. A very high negative predictive value (>95%) of coronary CT angiography reliably rules out the presence of significant CAD and can be used as a highly effective gatekeeper for invasive coronary angiography [91-93]. Thus, the need for further imaging examinations will only be restricted to those patients with an abnormal findings on coronary CT angiography. Consequently, the use of coronary CT angiography could avoid unnecessary invasive coronary angiography in most patients. This concept is also supported by relevant data about cost-effectiveness. Min *et al* investigated the value of coronary CT angiography as a first line test compared to myocardial perfusion imaging using single photon emission computed tomography (SPECT) in patients with a low to intermediate pre-test likelihood [94]. They concluded that lower referral rates to invasive coronary angiography and lower healthcare costs were observed in their low-risk group.

Figure 12.1 shows the diagnostic imaging pathways with use of coronary CT angiography and other imaging modalities in patients from different risk groups (pre-test probability of CAD). It is expected that the recommended pathways will assist physicians to appropriately choose coronary CT angiography in the diagnosis of patients with suspected CAD.

12.5.3. When Should Coronary CT Angiography Be Referred for Risk Stratification?

Coronary CT angiography is one of the most exciting developments in recent years in the diagnosis of CAD. The use of both non-invasive and invasive studies has increased substantially, and the cost of imaging services has doubled from 2000 to 2006 according to the Government report in the United States [95], with $14.1 billion in Medicare spending for imaging services ((www.gao.gov/products/ GAO-08-452). The increased use of non-invasive imaging should aim for more effective risk stratification of patients, allowing identification of those patients who would be most likely to benefit from invasive coronary angiography and ideally reduce the number of invasive procedure in patients who do not have obstructive disease. Thus, the key role of coronary CT angiography has to be defined clearly by physicians (mainly the cardiologists) as to when this technique is appropriately selected for diagnostic purposes. However, current clinical and imaging algorithms are suboptimal with regard to the proper identification of patients with obstructive CAD and judicious use of coronary CT angiography as a risk stratification approach [96].

In the ACCURACY trial which involved 230 patients with typical angina or atypical chest pain who were referred from 16 centers for invasive coronary angiography, 75.2% of the patients had normal coronary arteries or non-obstructive CAD on invasive coronary angiography [12]. Kim *et al* in their literature review indicated that up to 10% of patients thought to have ST-elevation myocardial infarction and up to 32% of patients thought to have acute coronary syndrome had normal coronary arteries or non-obstructive disease on invasive coronary angiography [97]. Patel *et al* in their study consisting of 398,978 patients who had undergone invasive coronary angiography reported that 62.4% had either normal coronary arteries or non-obstructive CAD (≤50% stenosis) [98]. Among those with a positive non-invasive test result, 58.7% had either no disease or non-obstructive CAD on invasive coronary angiography; whereas among those with negative non-invasive test results, 28.3% were in fact found to have obstructive CAD. These studies suggest that many unnecessary invasive coronary angiography examinations were performed in the clinical evaluation of patients with suspected CAD. Coronary CT angiography is an effective imaging modality of determining which patients should proceed to invasive coronary angiography.

Appropriate criteria for coronary CT angiography have been developed in 2006 by a multidisciplinary task force [99]. These criteria are well known and appear to be used by many practicing physicians. It is recommended that coronary CT angiography be appropriate in patients with chest pain syndrome who had an intermediate pretest probability of CAD, or in chest pain syndrome patients with an uninterpretable or equivocal stress test. A list of indications that were thought to be of uncertain appropriateness as well as a list of indications for which coronary CT angiography was considered inappropriate has been provided in the document. Due to rapid technological developments of multislice CT, researchers expressed concern about the "exploding use" of coronary CT angiography and that we do not yet know enough about how it changes patient management or leads to better outcomes [100, 101].

However, a recent study has reported that coronary CT angiography is actually underutilized when compared to myocardial perfusion imaging (MPI). Levin *et al* assessed utilization trends of coronary CT angiography and determined how rapidly this relative new procedure is growing over a 10-year period study [102]. Their results showed that although coronary CT angiography and MPI are useful imaging modalities in the diagnosis of suspected CAD and often provide complementary information, there were 44 times as many MPI as coronary CT angiography examinations in 2008. As a widely publicized technology, coronary CT angiography underwent a phase of rapid growth during its early years, but it declined in use in 2008, according to Levin et al's findings. Their observation emphasizes that invasive coronary angiography and MPI are over utilized, while coronary CT angiography is the procedure that should be recommended with greater use in an effort to more definitely determine the severity of disease in patients with suspected CAD and to reduce the use of invasive and expensive procedures. The diagnostic pathways with regard to appropriate use of coronary CT angiography for risk stratification in patients with suspected CAD are shown in Figure 12.1.

Conclusion

Coronary CT angiography has become an important non-invasive imaging modality in the diagnosis of suspected CAD. The technological advances in multislice CT gradually overcome the above-mentioned technical and diagnostic challenges, thus, these advances have a dramatic impact on its accuracy to diagnose CAD. The role of coronary CT angiography will continue to grow with wide availability of multislice CT scanner and its improved capabilities. However, the need for any given cardiac CT examination should always be justified on the basis of the individual patient's benefits and risks, given the fact that CT is an imaging modality associated with high radiation dose. Accurate risk stratification for appropriate selection of diagnostic methods of CAD is crucial, and both radiologists and referring physicians need to work together to develop better selection criteria for patients referred for coronary CT angiography. The main purpose of utilizing coronary CT angiography is to address specific clinical questions without allowing concerns about radiation exposure to dissuade physicians or their patients from obtaining or undergoing the required examination.

References

[1] Lloyd-Jones D, Adams RJ, Brown TM, et al. Executive summary: heart disease and stoke statistics 2010 update: A report from the American Heart Association. *Circulation* 2010; 121: 948-954.

[2] Gaziano TA, Bitton A, Anand S, Abrahams-Gessel S, Murphy A. Growing epidemic of coronary heart disease in low-and middle-income countries. *Curr Probl Cardiol* 2010; 35: 72-115.

[3] WHO. The World Health Report 2002: Reducing Risks, Promoting Healthy Life. Geneva: World Health Organization, 2002.

[4] http://www.who.int/whostat2007/en/index.html).

[5] Noto TJ Jr, Johnson LW, Krone R, et al. Cardiac catheterization 1990: a report of the registry of the Society for Cardiac Angiography and Interventions. (SCA&I). *Cathet Cardiovasc Diagn* 1991; 24:75–83.

[6] Fayad ZA, Fuster V, Nikolaou K, Becker C. Computed tomography and magnetic resonance imaging for non-invasive coronary artery and plaque imaging: current and potential future concepts. *Circulation* 2002; 106:2026–34.

[7] Lipton M, Higgins CB, Boyd DP. Computed tomography of the heart: evaluation of anatomy and function. *J Am Coll Cardiol* 1985; 5(Suppl.): S55–S69.

[8] McCollough CH, Zink FE. Performance evaluation of a multi-slice CT system. *Med Phys* 1999; 26:2223–30.

[9] Nieman K, Oudkerk M, Rensing BJ, et al. Coronary angiography with multi-slice computed tomography. *Lancet* 2001; 357:599–603.

[10] Sun Z, Lin CH, Davidson R, et al. Diagnostic value of 64-slice CT angiography in coronary artery disease: A systematic review. *Eur J Radiol* 2008; 67: 78-84.

[11] Miller JM, Rochitte CE, Dewey M, et al. Diagnostic performance of coronary angiography by 64-row CT. *N Engl J Med* 2008; 359: 2324-2336.

[12] Budoff MJ, Dowe D, Jollis JG, et al. Diagnostic performance of 64-multidetector row coronary computed tomographic angiography for evaluation of coronary artery stenosis in individuals without known coronary artery disease: results from the prospective multicenter ACCURACY (Assessment by Coronary Computed Tomographic Angiography of Individuals Undergoing Invasive Coronary Angiography) trial. *J Am Coll Cardiol* 2008;52:1724-1732.

[13] Meijboom WB, Meijs MFL, Schuijf JD, et al. Diagnostic accuracy of 64-slice computed tomography coronary angiography: a prospective multicenter, multivendor study. *J Am Coll Cardiol* 2008; 52:2135-2144.

[14] Min JK, Feignouz J, Treutenaere J, et al. The prognostic value of multidetector coronary CT angiography for the prediction of major adverse cardiac events: a major multicenter observational cohort study. *Int J Cardiovasc Imaging* 2010; 26: 721-728.

[15] Abdulla J, Asferg C, Kofoed KF. Prognostic value of absence or presence of coronary artery disease determined by 64-slice computed tomography coronary angiography: a systematic review and meta-analysis. *Int J Cardiovasc Imaging* 2011; 27: 413-420.

[16] De Roos A, Kroft LJ, Bax JJ, Lamb HJ, Geleijns J. Cardiac applications of multislice computed tomography. *Br J Radiol* 2006; 79:9-16.

[17] Roberts TW, Bax JJ, Davies LC. Cardiac CT and CT coronary angiography: technology and application. *Heart* 2008; 94:781-792.

[18] Achenbach S, Ropers D, Holle J, Muschiol G, Daniel WG, Moshage W. In-plane coronary arterial motion velocity: measurement with electron-beam CT. *Radiology* 2000; 216:457–463.

[19] Sun Z, Choo GH, Ng KH. Coronary CT angiography: current status and continuing challenges. *Br J Radiol* 2012; 85: 495-510.

[20] Sun Z, Jiang W. Diagnostic value of multislice CT angiography in coronary artery disease: A meta-analysis. *Eur J Radiol* 2006; 60: 279-286.

[21] Vanhoenacker PK, Heijenbrok-Kal MH, Van Heste R, et al. Diagnostic performance of multidetector CT angiography for assessment of coronary artery disease: meta-analysis. *Radiology* 2007; 244: 419-428.

[22] Abdulla J, Abildstrom Z, Gotzsche O, Christensen E, Kober L, Torp-Pedersen C. 64-multislice detector computed tomography coronary angiography as potential alternative to conventional coronary angiography: a systematic review and meta-analysis. *Eur Heart J* 2007; 28: 3042-3050.

[23] Mowatt G, Cook JA, Hillis GS, et al. 64-slice computed tomography angiography in the diagnosis and assessment of coronary artery disease: systematic review and meta-analysis. *Heart* 2008; 94: 1386–1393.

[24] Stein PD, Yaekoub AY, Matta F, Sostman HD. 64-slice CT for diagnosis of coronary artery disease: a systematic review. *Am J Med* 2008; 121: 715-725.

[25] Doninno R, Jacobs JE, Doshi JV, et al. Dual-source versus single-source cardiac CT angiography: comparison of diagnostic image quality. *AJR Am J Roentgenol* 2009; 192:1051-1056.

[26] Fang XM, Chen HW, Hu XY, et al. Dual-source CT coronary angiography without heart rate or rhythm control in comparison with conventional coronary angiography. *Int J Cardiovasc Imaging* 2010; 26: 323-331.

[27] Ropers U, Ropers D, Pflederer T, et al. Influence of heart rate on the diagnostic accuracy of dual-source computed tomography coronary angiography. *J Am Coll Cardiol* 2007; 50: 2393-2398.

[28] Leber AW, Johnson T, Becker A, et al. Diagnostic accuracy of dual-source multi-slice CT coronary angiography in patients with an intermediate pretest likelihood for coronary artery disease. *Eur Heart J* 2007; 28: 2354-2360.

[29] Scheffel H, Stolzmann P, Alkadhi H, et al. Low-dose CT and cardiac MR for the diagnosis of coronary artery disease: accuracy of single and combined approaches. *Int J Cardiovasc Imaging* 2010; 26: 579-590.

[30] LaBounty TM, Leipsic J, Mancini J, et al. Effect of a standardized radiation dose reduction protocol on diagnostic accuracy of coronary computed tomographic angiography. *Am J Cardiol* 2010; 106: 287-292.

[31] de Graaf FR, Schuijf JD, van Velzen JE, et al. Diagnostic accuracy of 320-row multidetector computed tomography coronary angiography in the non-invasive evaluation of significant coronary artery disease. *Eur Heart J* 2010; 31: 1908-1915.

[32] Donati OF, Stolzmann P, Desbiolles L, et al. Coronary artery disease: which degree of coronary artery stenosis is indicative of ischemia? *Eur J Radiol* 2011; 80: 120-126.

[33] Committee to Assess Health Risks from Exposure to Low Levels of Ionizing Radiation; Nuclear and Radiation Studies Board, Division on Earth and Life Studies, National Research Council of the National Academies. *Health Risks From Exposure to Low Levels of Ionizing Radiation:* BEIR VII Phase 2. Washington, DC: The National Academies Press; 2006.

[34] Brenner DJ, Hall EJ. Computed tomography—an increasing source of radiation exposure. *N Engl J Med* 2007; 357(22):2277–2284.

[35] Davies HE, Wathen CG, Gleeson FV. Risks of exposure to radiological imaging and how to minimise them. *BMJ* 2011; 342: 589-593.

[36] Smith-Bindman R, Lipson J, Marcus R, et al. Radiation dose associated with common computed tomography examinations and the associated lifetime attributable risk of cancer. *Arch Intern Med* 2009; 169: 2078-2086.

[37] Valentin J. The 2007 recommendations of the International Commission on Radiological Protection 103. *Annals of the ICRP* 2007;37:1-332.

[38] Gosling O, Loader R, Venables P, Rowles N, Morgan-Hughes G, Roobottom C. Cardiac CT: are we under-estimating the dose? A radiation dose study utilising the 2007 ICRP tissue weighting factors and a cardiac specific scan volume. *Clin Radiol* 2010; 65: 1013-1017.

[39] Einstein AJ, Elliston CD, Arai AE, et al. Radiation dose from single-heartbeat coronary CT angiography performed with a 320-detector row volume scanner. *Radiology* 2010; 254:698-706.

[40] Sun Z, Ng KH. Prospective versus retrospective ECG-gated multislice CT coronary angiography: A systematic review of radiation dose and diagnostic accuracy. *Eur J Radiol* 2012; 81: e94-e100.

[41] Paul JF, Abada HT. Strategies for reduction of radiation dose in cardiac multislice CT. *Eur Radiol* 2007; 17:2028-2037.

[42] Hausleiter J, Meyer T, Hermann F, et al. Estimated radiation dose associated with cardiac CT angiography. *JAMA* 2009; 301(5):500–507.

[43] Haaga JR. Radiation dose management: weighing risk versus benefit. *AJR Am J Roentgenol* 2001; 177(2):289–91.

[44] Golding SJ, Shrimpton PC. Commentary. Radiation dose in CT: are we meeting the challenge? *Br J Radiol* 2002;75(889):1–4.

[45] Report of the United Nations Scientific Committee on the Effects of Atomic Radiation. General Assembly Official Records. 63rd Session. Suppl 46. 2008. www.undemocracy.com/A-63-398.pdf.

[46] Dewey M, Zimmermann E, Deissenrieder F, et al. Noninvasive coronary angiography by 320-row computed tomography with lower radiation exposure and maintained diagnostic accuracy: Comparisons of results with cardiac catheterization in a head-to-head pilot investigation. *Circulation* 2009; 120: 867-875.

[47] Balter S, Zanzonico P, Reiss GP, Moses JW. Radiation is not the only risk. *AJR J Roentgenol* 2011; 196: 762-767.

[48] Tubiana M. Computed tomography and radiation exposure. *N Engl J Med* 2008; 358:850, author reply 852–853.

[49] Schwartz DT. Counter-point: are we really ordering too many CT scans? *West J Emerg Med* 2008; 9:120–122.

[50] Thomas KE, Parnell-Parmley JE, Haidar S, et al. Assessment of radiation dose awareness among pediatricians. *Pediatr Radiol* 2006;36:823–32.

[51] Lee CI, Haims AH, Monico EP, Brink JA, Forman HP. Diagnostic CT scans: assessment of patient, physician, and radiologist awareness of radiation dose and possible risks. *Radiology* 2004;231:393–8.

[52] Jacob K, Vivian G, Steel JR. X-ray dose training: are we exposed to enough? *Clin Radiol* 2004; 59:928–34.

[53] Heyer CM, Hansmann J, Peters SA, Lemburg SP. Paediatrician awareness of radiation dose and inherent risks in chest imaging studies—a questionnaire study. *Eur J Radiol* 2010; 76: 288-293.

[54] Shiralkar S, Rennie A, Snow M, et al. Doctors' knowledge of radiation exposure: questionnaire study. *BMJ* 2003; 327: 371-372.

[55] Krille L, Hammer GP, Merzenich H, Zeeb H. Systematic reveiw on physicians' knowledge about radiation doses and radiation risks of computed tomography. *Eur J Radiol* 2010; 76: 36-41.

[56] Wong CS, Huang BS, Sin HK, Wong WL, Yiu KL, Chu Y. A questionnaire study assessing local physicians, radiologist and interns' knowledge and practivce pertaining to radiation exposure related to radiological imaigng, *Eur J Radiol* 2012; 81: e264-e268.

[57] van den Brink-Muinen A, van Dulmen SM, de Haes HCJM, Visser AP, Schellevis FG, Bensing JM. Has patients' involvement in the decision-making process changed over time? *Health Expect* 2006;9(4):333-342.

[58] Degner LF, Kristjanson LJ, Bowman D, et al. Information need and decisional preferences in women with breast cancer. *JAMA* 1997;277(18):1485-1492.

[59] Caoili EM, Cohan RH, Ellis JH, et al. Medical decision making regarding computed tomographic radiation dose and associated risk: The patient's perspective. *Arch Intern Med* 2009; 169:1069-1071.

[60] Dauer L, Thornton RH, Hay JL, Balter R, Williamson MJ, Germain J. Fears, feelings, and facts: interactively communicating benefits and risks of medical radiation with patients. *AJR Am J Roentgenol* 2011; 196: 756-761.

[61] Larson DB, Rader SB, Forman HP, Fenton LZ. Informing parents about CT radiation exposure in children: it's ok to tell them. *AJR Am J Roentgenol* 2007;189: 271-5.

[62] RCP Working Party. Making the Best Use of a Department of Clinical Radiology Services: *Referral Guidelines.* 6th ed. London: The Royal College of Radiologists; 2007.

[63] Meijboom WB, van Mieghem CA, Mollet NR, et al. 64-slice computed tomography coronary angiography in patients with high, intermediate, or low pretest probability of significant coronary artery disease. *J Am Coll Cardiol* 2007; 50: 1469-1475.

[64] Greenland P, Bonow RO, Brundage BH, et al. ACCF/AHA 2007 clinical expert consensus document on coronary artery calcium scoring by computed tomography in global cardiovascular risk assessment and in evaluation of patients with chest pain: a report of the American College of Cardiology Foundation Clinical Expert Consensus Task Force (ACCF/AHA Writing Committee to Update the 2000 Expert Consensus Document on Electron Beam Computed Tomography). *Circulation* 2007; 115:402–426.

[65] Oudkerk M, Stillman AE, Halliburton SS, et al. Coronary artery calcium screening: current status and recommendations from the European Society of Cardiac Radiology and North American Society for Cardiovascular Imaging. *Int J Cardiovasc Imaging* 2008; 24:645–671.

[66] Hoffmann U, Siebert U, Bull-Stewart A, et al. Evidence for lower variability of coronary artery calcium mineral mass measurements by multidetector computed tomography in a community based cohort-consequences for progression studies. *Eur J Radiol* 2006; 57:396–402.

[67] Haberl R, Becker A, Leber A, et al. Correlation of coronary calcification and angiographically documented stenoses in patients with suspected coronary artery disease: results of 1,764 patients. *J Am Coll Cardiol* 2001;37:451– 457.

[68] Ostrom MP, Gopal A, Ahmadi N, et al. Mortality incidence and the severity of coronary atherosclerosis assessed by computed tomography angiography. *J Am Coll Cardiol* 2008; 52: 1335-1343.

[69] Detrano R, Guerci AD, Carr JJ, et al. Coronary calcium as a predictor of coronary events in four racial or ethnic groups. *N Engl J Med* 2008; 358: 1336 –1345.

[70] Budoff MJ, Shaw LJ, Liu ST, et al. Long-term prognosis associated with coronary calcification: observations from a registry of 25,253 patients. *J Am Coll Cardiol* 2007; 49: 1860 – 1870.

[71] Shaw LJ, Raggi P, Schisterman E, Berman DS, Callister TQ. Prognostic value of cardiac risk factors and coronary artery calcium screening for all-cause mortality. *Radiology* 2003; 228: 826 – 833.

[72] Rubinshtein R, Gaspar T, Halon DA, et al. Prevalence and extent of obstructive coronary artery disease in patients with zero or low calcium score undergoing 64-slice cardiac multidetector computed tomography for evaluation of a chest pain syndrome. *Am J Cardiol* 2007; 99:472–475.

[73] van der Bijl N, Joemai RMS, Geleijns J, et al. Assessment of Agatston coronary artery calcium score using contrast-enhanced CT coronary angiography. *AJR Am J Roentgenol* 2010; 195: 1299-1305.

[74] van Werkhoven JM, Shuijf JD, Gaemperli O, et al. Incremental prognostic value of multi-slice computed tomography coronary angiography over coronary artery calcium scoring in patients with suspected coronary artery disease. *Eur Heart J* 2009; 30: 2622-2629.

[75] Kwon SW, Kim YJ, Shim J, et al. Coronary artery calcium scoring does not add prognostic value to standard 64-section CT angiography protocol in low-risk patients suspected of having coronary artery disease. *Radiology* 2011; 259: 92-99.

[76] American Heart Assocation, Clinical expert consensus document on coronary artery calcium scoring by computed tomography in global cardiovascular risk assessment and in evaluation of patients with chest pain, ACCF/AHA 2007, *Circulation* 2007;115: 402–426.

[77] O'Rourke R, Brundage BH, Froelicher VF, et al., American College of Cardiology/American Heart Association expert consensus document on electron beam computed tomography for the diagnosis and prognosis of coronary artery disease, *Circulation* 2000; 102:326–140.

[78] Cardiac Society of Australia and New Zealand, High speed computed tomography to detect coronary calcification, position statement from the cardiac society of Australia and New Zealand, www.csanz.edu.au/news/ inthenews/highspeed_ computer_tomography.pdf

[79] US Preventive Services Task Force, Screening for coronary heart disease, http//www.ahrq.gov/clinic/uspstf/uspscad.htm.

[80] De Backer G, Ambrosioni E, Borch-Johnson K, et al., European guidelines on cardiovascular disease prevention in clinical practice, Third Joint Task Force of European and other Societies on Cardiovascular Disease Prevention in Clinical Practice (constituted by representatives of eight societies and by invited experts), *Eur Heart J* 2003; 24: 1601–1610.

[81] Silber S, Richartz BM. Impact of both cardiac CT and cardiac MR on the assessment of cardiac risk, *Z. Kardiol.* 94 Suppl. 4:IV (2005) 70–80.

[82] Efstathopoulos EP, Pantos I, Thalassinou S, et al. Patient radiation doses in cardiac computed tomography: comparison of published results with prospective and retrospective acquisition. *Radiat Prot Dosim* 2012; 148: 83-91.
[83] Gottlieb I, Miller JM, Arbab-Zadeh A, et al. The absence of coronary calcification does not exclude obstructive coronary artery disease or the need for revascularization in patients referred for conventional coronary angiography. *J Am Coll Cardiol* 2010, 55:627–634.
[84] Chang SM, Nabi F, Xu J, et al. The coronary artery calcium score and stress myocardial perfusion imaging provide independent and complementary prediction of cardiac risk. *J Am Coll Cardiol* 2009, 54:1872–1882.
[85] Lau GT, Ridley LJ, Schieb MC, et al. Coronary artery stenoses: detection with calcium scoring, CT angiography, and both methods combined. *Radiology* 2005, 235:415–422.
[86] Cheng VY, Lepor NE, Madyoon H, et al. Presence and severity of noncalcified coronary plaque on 64-slice computed tomographic coronary angiography in patients with zero and low coronary artery calcium. *Am J Cardiol* 2007; 99:1183–1186.
[87] Hausleiter J, Meyer T, Hadamitzky M, et al. Prevalence of noncalcified coronary plaques by 64-slice computed tomography in patients with an intermediate risk for significant coronary artery disease. *J Am Coll Cardiol* 2006; 48: 312-318.
[88] Akram K, O'Donnell RE, King S, et al. Influence of symptomatic status on the prevalence of obstructive coronary artery disease in patients with zero calcium score. *Atherosclerosis* 2009; 203: 533-537.
[89] Nasis A, Leung MC, Antonis PR, et al. Diagnostic accuracy of non-invasive coronary angiography with 320-detector row computed tomography. *Am J Cardiol* 2010; 106: 1429-1435.
[90] Al Moudi M, Sun Z, Lenzo N. Diagnostic value of SPECT, PET and PET/CT in the diagnosis of coronary artery disease: A systematic review. *Biomed Imaging Interv J* 2011; 7 (2): e9.
[91] van Werkhoven JM, Gaemperli O, Schuijf JD, et al. Multislice computed tomography coronary angiography for risk stratification in patients with an intermediate pretest likelihood. *Heart* 2009; 95: 1607-1611.
[92] Leber AW, Johnson T, Becker A, et al. Diagnostic accuracy of dual-source multi-slice CT-coronary angiography in patients with an intermediate pretest likelihood for coronary artery disease. *Eur Heart J* 2007;28:2354 –2360.
[93] van Werkhoven JM, Heijenbrok MW, Schuijf JD, et al. Diagnostic accuracy of 64-slice multislice computed tomographic coronary angiography in patients with an intermediate pretest likelihood for coronary artery disease. *Am J Cardiol* 2010; 105: 302-305.
[94] Min JK, Kang N, Shaw LJ, et al. Costs and clinical outcomes after coronary multidetector CT angiography in patients without known coronary artery disease: comparison to myocardial perfusion SPECT. *Radiology* 2008;249:62–70.
[95] Lucas FL, DeLorenzo MA, Siewers AE, Wennberg DE. Temporal trends in the utilization of diagnostic testing and treatments for cardiovascular disease in the United States, 1993-2001. *Circulation* 2006; 113:374-9.
[96] Min JK, Shaw LJ, Berman DS. The present state of coronary computed tomography angiography: a process in evolution. *J Am Coll Cardiol* 2010; 55:957–965.

[97] Kim HW, Farzaneh-Far A, Kim RJ. Cardiovascular magnetic resonance in patients with myocardial infarction: current and emerging applications. *J Am Coll Cardiol* 2009; 55:1–16.

[98] Patel MR, Peterson ED, Dai D, et al. Low diagnostic yield of elective coronary angiography. *N Engl J Med* 2010; 362:886–895.

[99] Hendel RC, Patel MR, Kramer CM, et al. ACCF/ ACR/SCCT/SCMR/ASNC /NASCI/SCAI/SIR 2006 appropriateness criteria for cardiac computed tomography and cardiac magnetic resonance imaging. *J Am Coll Cardiol* 2006; 48:1475–1497.

[100] Redberg RF, Walsh J. Pay now, benefits may follow: the case of cardiac computed tomographic angiography. *N Engl J Med* 2008; 359:2309–2311.

[101] Redberg RF. Computed tomographic angiography: more than just a pretty picture? *J Am Coll Cardiol* 2007; 49:1827–1829.

[102] Levin DC, Parker L, Halpern EJ, Julsrud PR, Rao VM. The lack of growth in use of coronary CT angiograhy: Is it being approriately used? *AJR Am J Roentgenol* 2011; 196: 862-867.

Chapter 13

Coronary CT Angiography in Coronary Artery Disease: Summary and Conclusion

The recent technological developments in cardiac CT provide the ability to examine the cardiac structure with a level of detail that was not previously possible. Coronary CT angiography represents the most rapidly developed imaging modality in cardiac imaging, with satisfactory results having been achieved in the diagnosis of coronary artery disease. The technological advances in multislice CT from 4- to 64- and to 320-slice scanners have gradually overcome the technical and diagnostic challenges, resulting in better quality of cardiac images. Thus, these advances have a dramatic impact on its accuracy in diagnosis of coronary artery disease. The role of coronary CT angiography will continue to grow with the wide availability of multislice CT scanners and its improved capabilities.

Coronary CT angiography demonstrates high accuracy for detection and characterization of atherosclerotic plaques, evaluation of coronary stenosis and accurate prediction of major adverse cardiac events. Thus, coronary CT angiography could serve as a reliable imaging modality to predict atherosclerosis and prevent further development of coronary artery disease.

Although coronary CT angiography cannot fully replace invasive coronary angiography in diagnosis of coronary artery disease, it could serve as an effective and independent predictor for predicting coronary artery disease progress and major cardiac events. This has significant clinical value because a normal coronary CT angiography suggests that patients who have normal coronary arteries and can be safely reassured without undergoing further tests or invasive examinations such as invasive coronary angiography.

Radiation dose becomes an issue for coronary CT angiography mainly due to low pitch values required for acquisition of gapless cardiac images and special image reconstruction process. Radiation dose associated with coronary CT angiography has increased substantially over the last decade with the development of multislice CT scanners and widespread use of CT technique in cardiac imaging. This has raised serious concerns, which need to be drawn to the attention of both clinicians and manufacturers. However, several steps can be taken to reduce the dose, with very effective outcomes having been achieved, as discussed in the previous chapters. With application of appropriate dose-saving strategies, coronary CT angiography dose is approximately equivalent to or even lower than that of an invasive coronary angiography.

Tremendous progress has been made to reduce the radiation dose; however, much effort is still required to ensure that coronary CT angiography is safely performed in imaging patients with suspected coronary artery disease. Accurate risk stratification for appropriate selection of coronary CT angiography is crucial, and both radiologists and referring physicians (mainly cardiologists) need to work together to develop better selection criteria for patients referred for coronary CT angiography. Utilization of coronary CT angiography must be defined as to whether it leads to the greatest benefit and whether the radiation risk may be greater than the benefit expected from the CT examinations.

Index

D

E

M

N

O

P

Q

R

S

T

U

V

W

Y